CNOR Exam Study Guide & Practice Resource

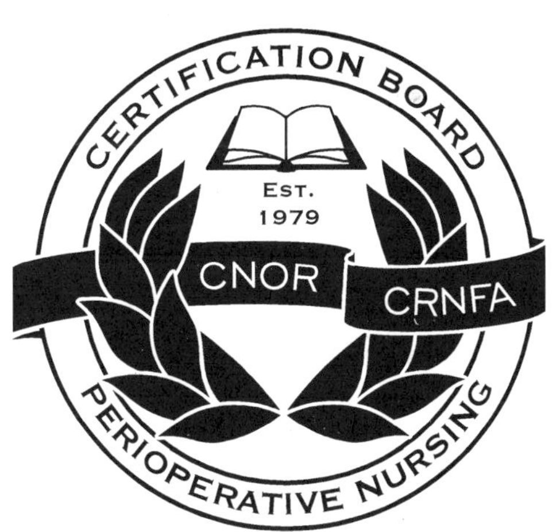

Published by
Certification Board Perioperative Nursing
2170 South Parker Road, Suite 295
Denver, CO 80231

CNOR™ Exam Study Guide & Practice Resource

Content Coordinator:

Dru Beedle, RN, MN, CNOR, CNA

Published by:

Certification Board Perioperative Nursing

This study guide has been developed in an effort to provide information for the perioperative nurse who is preparing for the CNOR examination. The perioperative nurse's scope of practice has been used as the overall basis for the organization of this publication and also serves as the basic framework for each chapter.

The Certification Board Perioperative Nursing presents this publication in the hope that it will serve to enhance the knowledge and skill level of the perioperative nurse who strives to demonstrate professional achievement in practice.

Printed in the United States of America

ISBN 0-9717619-1-4

TABLE OF CONTENTS

PREFACE

This examination resource guide is meant to function as one of several tools that will help you reach your goal of CNOR certification. The chapters in this book correlate with the Job Analysis and Test Specifications. The Job Analysis describes the overall functions and responsibilities as well as the underlying knowledge and skills that are essential to ensure proficiency as a perioperative nurse. The Test Specifications are guidelines used for developing the certification examination.

The chapter titles of chapters one through 16 indicate task statements from the Job Analysis. A task statement is a component of the Job Analysis that describes work activities that an entry-level perioperative nurse may perform. Within each chapter are knowledge and skill statements. Knowledge statements describe an organized body of information, usually of a factual or procedural nature. When applied, a knowledge statement makes successful performance of the task statement possible. A skill statement describes the proficient manual, verbal, or mental manipulation of data, people, or things. Skills embody observable, quantifiable, and measurable performance characteristics.

At the end of each chapter is a list of Recommended Study Material. After identifying the area in which you might need additional help, you may want to refer to the resources listed to assist in preparing for the exam. The examination is constructed to reflect the professional actions taken by perioperative nurses in providing care for patients during the preoperative, intraoperative, and postoperative period. Questions test a candidate's ability to apply knowledge and skills to practice.

Chapter 17, "Strategies for Success: Getting Prepared and Being Test-Wise," provides information about planning a personalized study program. You will find information on the processes involved with answering multiple-choice test questions and developing skills in test-taking strategies. This chapter provides the candidate with tools on how to be successful in passing the CNOR certification examination.

You may find it helpful to form a study group and use this book as a template to plan study sessions. Statistics show that people retain more information when they read it, verbalize it, and write it, than when it is simply read.

If you have questions about this study resource guide, please contact the Director of Certification at the Certification Board Perioperative Nursing at 888-257-2667.

Good luck as you embark on this exciting phase of your career.

Mary Leaven O'Neale, RN, MN, CNOR
Director of Certification
Certification Board Perioperative Nursing

CONTRIBUTING AUTHORS

Dru A. Beedle, RN, MN, CNOR, CNA
Consultant
Lindenhurst, Illinois

Linda Brazen, RN, MSN, CNOR
Clinical Director
The Children's Hospital
Denver, Colorado

Robin Chard, RN, MSN, CNOR
Assistant Professor, School of Nursing
Florida International University
Miami, Florida

Brenda S. Gregory Dawes, RN, MSN, CNOR
Innovations Liaison
Sandel Medical Industries
New Port Richey, Florida

Georgia Dinndorf, RN, BSN, CNOR
Surgery Staff Nurse
St. Cloud Hospital
St. Cloud, Minnesota

Janess Dulinski, RN, MSN, CNOR
Orthopedic Team Leader
Illinois Masonic Medical Center
Chicago, Illinois

Sylvia Durrance, RN, BSN, CNOR
Clinical Manager
California Pacific Medical Center
San Francisco, California

Nancymarie Fortunato-Phillips, RN, BSN, MEd, CNOR, CPSN
Perioperative Nursing Educator
Lakeland Community College
Kirkland, Ohio

Linda K. Groah, RN, MS, CNOR, CNAA, FAAN
Chief Operating Officer
Kaiser Foundation Hospital
San Francisco, California

Susan Renée Guerra, RN, MN, CNOR, CNAA
Business Process Review Manager
Siemens Healthcare Services
London, England

Cynthia K. Halvorson, RN, MSN, CNOR
Consultant
Englewood, Colorado

Julia M. Leahy, RN, PhD
Principal and Director, Test Development
The Chauncey Group International
Princeton, New Jersey

Rose Moss, RN, MN, CNOR
Senior Account Manager
HealthStream
Denver, Colorado

Rose Seavey, RN, MBA, CNOR, ACSP
Director of Sterile Processing
The Children's Hospital
Denver, Colorado

Carol A. Sparks, RN, BSN, CNOR
Manager, OR
University of Connecticut Health Center
Farmington, Connecticut

Linda D. Waters, RN, PhD
Managing Principal, Health & Professional Division
The Chauncey Group International
Princeton, New Jersey

Mary Lynne Weemering, RN, MSN, CNOR
Special Projects Coordinator
Kingwood, Texas

CHAPTER 1: ASSESS HEALTH STATUS OF PATIENT

Georgia Dinndorf, RN, BSN, CNOR

This chapter reviews the assessment of the health status of the perioperative patient. The first step in the nursing process is assessment. Health assessment occurs immediately upon the patient's decision to undergo surgery. Nursing assessment is not delegated to unlicensed personnel. The perioperative nurse formulates nursing diagnoses from the health assessment data. Collection of certain health assessment data can be delegated to a person with the appropriate training and skills to collect the data. For example, an unlicensed person may take the vital signs, and the professional registered nurse determines whether the vital signs are within normal limits. The perioperative nurse uses the North American Nursing Diagnosis Association (NANDA) nursing diagnoses to identify the patient's existing needs and risk potential. The perioperative nurse then uses nursing diagnoses to determine the nursing interventions and identify the expected outcomes. To effectively and efficiently assess the patient's health, the perioperative nurse should know

- what data to collect,
- where to locate data,
- how to collect the data,
- how to organize the data,
- how to analyze and interpret information, and
- how to formulate NANDA approved nursing diagnoses.

The perioperative nurse must be experienced in

- clinical observations,
- communication,
- physical assessment,
- decision making,
- inferential reasoning,
- conceptualization, and
- critical judgment.

The CNOR examination addresses the health assessment of the patient's surgical experience in the preoperative, intraoperative, and postoperative phases. This chapter will help perioperative nurses recognize their strengths and learning needs. This chapter includes the application of the skills to case studies and patient situations.

LEARNING OBJECTIVES

Upon completion of this chapter, the perioperative nurse will be able to:

1. Collect physiological, psychological, and psychosocial data.
2. Analyze data to formulate nursing diagnoses.
3. Develop nursing diagnoses to use in creating nursing interventions.
4. Assess patients in all three phases of the surgical experience.
5. Revise the plan of care based on the patient's changing status.
6. Reassess the patient's status on an ongoing basis.

TASK STATEMENT; AREAS OF KNOWLEDGE AND SKILL

Task Statement

Assess the health status of the patient in order to develop an individualized age specific plan of care by collecting, categorizing, and interpreting data (physical and psychosocial) from documented information, observation, patient/family interview, and other health care team members. Nursing diagnoses are derived from assessment data.

Areas of Knowledge

- K-1 Health assessment techniques
- K-2 Anatomy and physiology
- K-3 Pathophysiology
- K-4 Pharmacology and anesthetic agents
- K-5 Pain management
- K-7 Diagnostic procedures and results
- K-15 Risks for injury, including but not limited to, skin, positioning, and retained foreign body
- K-16 Emergency procedures (eg, CPR, MH)
- K-18 Defining characteristics of impending patient physiologic crisis
- K-20 Sociology (eg, cultural and ethnic influences, family patterns, spirituality and related practices)
- K-21 Communication theories and techniques
- K-23 Discharge planning
- K-25 *Perioperative Nursing Data Set* (PNDS)
- K-27 Microbiology and infection control
- K-28 Standard and transmission-based precautions
- K-39 Patient rights and responsibilities
- K-40 Legal responsibilities and implications for patient care
- K-41 Approved nursing diagnoses (eg, NANDA)
- K-42 Nursing research and evidence-based practice
- K-43 "ANA Code of Ethics for Nurses with Explications for Perioperative Nurses"
- K-44 Regulatory standards and voluntary guidelines
- K-45 AORN *Standards, Recommended Practices, and Guidelines*
- K-46 AORN position statements (eg, bloodborne pathogens, do-not-resuscitate orders [DNR])
- K-47 Principles of problem solving
- K-48 Quality improvement principles
- K-50 Defining characteristics of impaired individuals (eg, substance abuse, psychological disturbance, compromised performance)
- K-52 Defining characteristics of domestic abuse (eg, child, elder, partner/spouse)
- K-56 Implants (eg, handling, tracking, sterilization)

Areas of Skill

- S-1 Confirming patient identity, operative site, and procedure
- S-2 Collecting, analyzing, and prioritizing patient data
- S-3 Using health assessment techniques (eg, interview, observation, auscultation, palpation, percussion)
- S-4 Communicating effectively (verbal and nonverbal)
- S-6 Evaluating environment for discharge care
- S-7 Assessing and managing pain
- S-8 Assessing for potential abuse (eg, substance, domestic)
- S-9 Assessing readiness to learn, knowledge level, and preferred learning style
- S-10 Identifying barriers to learning
- S-11 Identifying risk of infection and injury
- S-12 Identifying cultural, spiritual, and ethnic issues in care
- S-13 Identifying age specific needs
- S-16 Applying *AORN Standards, Recommended Practices, and Guidelines*
- S-17 Applying the *Perioperative Nursing Data Set* (PNDS)
- S-20 Maintaining accurate patient records
- S-23 Applying regulatory standards and voluntary guidelines
- S-30 Documenting all relevant facts and data elements with appropriate terminology
- S-35 Maintaining the dignity, modesty, and privacy of the patient and protecting the confidentiality of patient information
- S-45 Monitoring physiological parameters
- S-46 Anticipating and evaluating the effects of pharmacological and anesthetic agents
- S-48 Detecting significant changes in the environment
- S-54 Recognizing impaired behavior in patients, family, and staff and responding appropriately
- S-60 Directing health care team members in emergency situations
- S-61 Performing basic life support and other emergency procedures
- S-62 Setting priorities
- S-65 Applying ethical principles
- S-67 Evaluating for signs and symptoms of injury
- S-70 Classifying the surgical wound

PREOPERATIVE HEALTH ASSESSMENT

Assessment begins with gathering data about the patient and concludes with the formation of nursing diagnoses. The critical components of health assessment in the preoperative phase are as follows.

Identify and Use Health Data Sources

- scheduled surgical procedure
- medical records
- patient interviews
- family/significant others
- surgeon's preference card
- x-rays, magnetic resonance imaging (MRI), computed tomography (CT) scan, studies
- other members of the health care team (eg, nursing colleagues in the nursing unit or emergency department, surgeon, anesthesia care provider, allied health care providers such as radiology technicians and emergency medical technicians)
- monitoring devices

Review Pertinent Medical Records

The patient's medical record serves as a tool of communication between health care team members. Competent perioperative nursing practice requires the nurse to verify the patient's identity, the patient's understanding of the procedure, advance directives, and consent for the procedure. The policy of the institution may require that these documents accompany the patient to the surgical suite. If documents are missing, the perioperative nurse should follow the institution's protocol for obtaining the required documents. Reviewing the medical record usually includes

- baseline vital signs;
- laboratory results (most common lab values: glucose, blood urea nitrogen [BUN], sodium [Na], calcium [Ca], complete blood count [CBC], chloride [Cl], carbon dioxide [CO_2]);
- previous surgical procedures;
- existing medical problems;
- allergies and adverse reactions to drugs or latex;
- presence of implantable devices (eg, defibrillator);
- age;
- weight; and
- psychosocial data of significance.

In selected patients, reviewing the following may be appropriate:

- coagulation values (ie, prothrombin time/partial thromboplastin time [PT/PTT], international normalized ratio [INR]);
- electrocardiogram (ECG) tracing and results;
- radiology reports; and
- pathology reports.

The perioperative nurse may not need to review all of the above records for every patient; exceptions may be trauma patients. There may not be time or the opportunity for informed consent from the patient or family. The medical diagnosis and scheduled surgical procedure provide clues with regard to the type of medical records to review. For example, an open reduction of an ankle fracture will require an x-ray of the fracture. The x-ray assists the health care team members to prepare for the surgical procedure equipment, supplies, and positioning. Research indicates that certain preoperative studies, in certain patient populations, do not meaningfully contribute to the patient's outcome. Knowing what to look for is an acquired skill based on knowledge of the patient, the patient's condition, the surgical procedure, and experience as a perioperative nurse.

The Patient/Family Interview

The patient and/or family interview should be conducted in a private environment. The nurse's general demeanor, including eye contact, posture, and physical gestures, sends messages to the patient and the family. The interview should always begin with an introduction and brief explanation of the nurse's role in the patient's care. Giving the appearance of a professional, credible nurse and behaving in a caring and sensitive fashion will reassure the patient and family that the nurse is concerned about the welfare of the patient.

During the interview, the perioperative nurse explains the preoperative phase and the intraoperative and postoperative typical routines. During the preoperative assessment, the nurse focuses on psychosocial and cultural factors, mental and emotional status, physical assessment, and educational needs. Preoperative education helps the patient alleviate some apprehension and stress they may be experiencing. The patient's cultural factors may influence how they respond to surgical intervention.

The patient interview serves to

- identify the patient,
- obtain physical data,
- assess current emotional status,
- provide ideas to coping with the present situation,
- verify the informed consent for the procedure,
- demonstrate the patient's understanding and perceptions of the procedure,
- obtain the patient's expectations of care,
- confirm the advance directive,
- identify pertinent psychosocial influences, and
- provide information and education to the patient and family.

The interview time is an opportunity to explore and verify any allergies or problems with previous procedures. It also is a time to note psychosocial influences in the patient's environment. Questioning by the perioperative nurse during the preoperative assessment is needed to fully explore areas that are pertinent to the surgical experience.

An example of an opening question during the interview before a scheduled right total knee arthroplasty is, "Mr. G, you're here for surgery on your right knee. Is that correct?" This question confirms several items of data: 1) identifies the patient, 2) confirms the operative site, and 3) confirms the patient's basic understanding of surgery. The interview process is a time to assess the patient's psychosocial status. There are some important patient considerations that may arise out of the interview process. One concern may be that the patient is a Jehovah Witness and may not want blood products administered during or after the procedure. Some facilities conduct a preoperative interview over the telephone and may find this information out significantly before the procedure so the entire health care team knows the patient's request before the patient is admitted to the surgical preoperative area.

Specific populations or situations may make the patient interview more challenging and even impossible. Trauma patients may not be able to be interviewed. A small child or infant will need a parent to be interviewed. A patient with Alzheimer's disease or moderate dementia may need a family member present for the interview.

The Focused Physical Assessment

The focused physical assessment is information pertinent for the patient's diagnosis, surgical procedure, and pre-existing conditions. The four elements of the physical assessment are inspection/observation, auscultation, palpation, and percussion. The nurse should be experienced in all four and know which to use for the focused assessment. All four techniques may not be necessary for every patient.

Developing Nursing Diagnoses

Nursing diagnoses have three parts:

- the nursing diagnosis,
- "related to" phrase, and
- defining characteristics.

Nursing diagnoses should be individualized. For example, a mentally challenged patient is scheduled for a total joint arthroplasty. A nursing diagnosis is, "Knowledge deficit related to surgical intervention." An elderly lady with fragile skin would have a nursing diagnosis of, "Risk for impaired skin integrity related to surgical positioning." Nursing interventions are based on the nursing diagnoses.

INTRAOPERATIVE HEALTH ASSESSMENT

The focus of health assessment in the intraoperative phase changes to "at this moment in time." Physical assessment becomes more focused. Patient interviews have limited value for the patient receiving a general anesthetic; however, the patient interview may play a larger role with the awake, nonsedated patient.

Intraoperative nursing diagnoses have two forms:

- the nurse must assess the patient's response to nursing interventions and

- the nurse may need to formulate additional nursing diagnoses because the health assessment data changes as surgery progresses.

Changes in the patient's health status may dictate modification of the original nursing diagnoses.

POSTOPERATIVE HEALTH ASSESSMENT

Health assessment in the postoperative phase is similar to that of the intraoperative phase, and "this moment in time" mentality is used. The perioperative nurse may use monitoring devices more heavily in this phase. The perioperative nurse should review the medical record, which now includes intraoperative information. Physical assessment in the postoperative phase is focused on responses to nursing interventions. The patient interview plays a larger role in the assessment of patients having local or regional anesthetics. Modifying existing diagnoses or formulating new ones in response to changes in health status is the focus in the postoperative nursing diagnosis formation. Some new postoperative diagnoses may be

- pain related to surgical incision,
- hypothermia related to surgical site exposure, and
- fluid volume deficit related to postoperative blood loss.

SUMMARY

This chapter reviewed the health assessment of the patient in all three phases of the patient's surgical experience. It compared the differences in each phase of the surgical experience. The key components of health assessment were emphasized:

- identifying and utilizing health data resources,
- patient/family interview,
- focused physical assessment, and
- formulating individualized nursing diagnoses.

CASE STUDY

Case Study: Mr. C

Mr. C is a 48-year-old builder who was electively admitted to the hospital two days ago for a radical prostatectomy with lymph node dissection secondary to recently diagnosed prostate cancer. His past medical history is significant only for a previous operation for open surgical repair of a torn rotator cuff, suffered in a fall seven years ago. He has no allergies and takes no chronic medications. His preoperative lab values show hemoglobin (Hgb) of 13.4, white blood cell (WBC) count 6300, platelets 216,000, potassium 4.2, BUN 15, and creatinine 0.9. He received a general anesthetic for the procedure, and an intrathecal morphine injection was administered for control of acute postoperative pain.

The procedure was ultimately successful, though the operative time was 545 minutes, and the blood loss was estimated at 3,700 mL, which necessitated transfusion of one unit of packed red blood cells. His immediate recovery was uneventful.

By postoperative day two, the patient complained of lower abdominal pain and tenderness at his incision, along with persistent nausea. Bowel sounds were absent, and he had a temperature of 100.8° F. Examination is pertinent for an area of redness at the lower end of his incision with purulent drainage. He is scheduled for irrigation and debridement of his wound dehiscence. His most recent lab values (from this morning) include Hgb 11.2, WBC 15,400, BUN 19, and potassium 4.6.

Points to Consider—Preoperative

Where would you look for the pertinent data for this patient prior to his entering the operating room?

- Medications that have been given are listed in the medication administration record (MAR), while those that are to be administered can be found in the preoperative orders.
- Lab values and results of other studies (eg, ECG, CT scans) can be found in the appropriate sections of the current chart. Old films may need to be obtained from radiology archives.

Are any of the lab values of concern?

- The elevated WBC, in addition to the fever, likely indicates a wound infection, although atelectasis and/or pneumonia or urinary tract infection (UTI) cannot be excluded. The elevated BUN may indicate mild dehydration. The hemoglobin is low due to intraoperative blood loss.

What additional supplies and/or equipment are likely to be needed in this case?

- Supplies for obtaining cultures and gram stain specimens.

- Packing material if the wound is to be left open.
- Drains.
- Retention sutures, abdominal binder, Kerlix-laced dressing closure if the patient's body habitus warrants.

What precautions should be taken before induction of anesthesia?

- H2 blockers, nonparticulate antacids, and metoclopramide may be helpful in decreasing the likelihood of significant aspiration.

Would nasogastric suctioning be useful in this case?

- Pro: decreases the volume of retained gastric contents.
- Con: presence of nasograstric tube (NGT) may act as a wick (ensures an incompetent gastroesophageal [GE] sphincter).
- Could remove NGT after emptying stomach, but will almost certainly need to be replaced, which may lead to unnecessary nasal/pharyngeal trauma.

Points to Consider—Intraoperative

After transfer to the operating bed and application of necessary monitors, the patient is preoxygenated and cricoid pressure is applied. The induction medications are given, and after loss of the lid reflex, the patient's eyes are taped for protection in anticipation of intubation.

What is cricoid pressure?

- The cricoid cartilage is the only cartilage in the upper airway that encircles the entire trachea. As such; it can be compressed against the esophagus by applying pressure to the anterior neck. It can be identified by palpating the V-shaped notch at the superior aspect of the thyroid cartilage, then moving caudad over the thyroid cartilage, the slightly depressed crico-thyroid membrane, and finally the firm cricoid cartilage. Pressure should be applied firmly, but not to the point of distorting the anatomy—if your fingers are getting fatigued, you're pressing too hard!

What is the purpose of cricoid pressure?

- As pressure is applied, the cartilaginous ring is displaced against the compressible esophagus, occluding the lumen and decreasing the likelihood of gastric contents ascending into the oropharynx.

While waiting for the paralytic agent to take effect, a large amount of greenish-brown fluid begins to stream from the patient's mouth and nose.

What is happening?

- Cricoid pressure is not foolproof. In spite of its application, gastric contents have made their way into the oropharynx and are threatening to enter the trachea.

What is the next step?

- To prevent or minimize the consequences of acid aspiration syndrome, control of the airway must be obtained as soon as possible. The anesthesia care provider may take several steps in an attempt to decrease the volume of aspirate that makes its way into the trachea, and the function of the circulating nurse is to provide whatever assistance is necessary. This may include passing suction and other instruments during attempted intubation, repositioning the bed (Trendelenberg position may be used to take advantage of gravity's effect, although it is possible that this will increase the amount of fluid coming up from the stomach), or calling for assistance.

Difficulty was encountered during laryngoscopy, and the endotracheal tube was placed in the esophagus. This is quickly recognized, but the duration of apnea has now caused a drop in the oxygen saturation (SaO_2) to the low 80s.

What is the next step?

- Some would advocate mask ventilation with 100% oxygen to restore SaO_2 to an acceptable level before another attempt at intubation. Others would argue that application of positive pressure ventilation with a face mask in an airway known to be filled with vomitus will merely push the toxic stomach contents further into the periphery of the lung, leading to serious consequences later. There is no good answer. If the anesthesia care provider feels that successful intubation is eminent, another attempt is reasonable. If further difficulty is likely, however, the mantra "Bad breath is better that no breath" applies, and mask ventilation should begin.

In this case, a second attempt resulted in success and the endotracheal tube was inserted in the patient's trachea under direct vision.

How can a tracheal position be confirmed?

- Auscultation of breath sounds.
- Absence of gurgling sounds when the stomach is auscultated.
- Condensation in the endotracheal tube (ETT) during the expiratory phase.

- Persistent presence of CO_2 in the expired gases (Gold Standard).
- Fiber-optic inspection.

Suctioning of the ETT produces only the greenish fluid, and administration of albuterol combined with positive end-expiratory pressure (PEEP) results in a gradual return of SaO_2 to 96%. The inspired oxygen concentration was weaned to 50% before the end of the procedure, with no worsening of the SaO_2. By the conclusion of the case, no further fluid could be suctioned from the ETT. Because no wheezes were audible and the patient met criteria for extubation, he was awakened and extubated in the operating room prior to transport to the PACU.

Points to Consider—Postoperative

Immediately postoperatively, the patient is somewhat drowsy, but seems comfortable and reasonably oriented.

What monitoring should be employed in the PACU?

- Routine postanesthesia monitoring includes SaO_2, noninvasive blood pressure (NIBP), temperature, and pulse. Frequent determination of level of consciousness, pain scores, and other components of the Aldrete scale also are noted.

Admission vitals are blood pressure (BP) 143/69, heart rate (HR) 104, respiratory rate (RR) 18, temperature 99.9° F, SaO_2 97% (on 50% face mask O_2).

Are any special tests or procedures indicated?

- A chest x-ray (CXR) should be obtained to provide a baseline for comparison should the patient's condition deteriorate. An arterial blood sample would be very helpful should his condition deteriorate.

CXR shows mild interstitial fluid throughout most of the lung, but no 'whited-out' areas.

What is the significance of a 'whited-out' area?

- A lung field with no ventilation will appear white on CXR. This indicates blockage of the airway. The patient may benefit from bronchoscopy, under the assumption that aspirated particulate matter from the stomach has caused obstruction of the bronchus.
- The presence of particulate matter in the aspirate correlates with a greater rate of complications in patients with acid aspiration syndrome. Other poor prognostic indicators are an aspirated volume of greater than 25 mL and an aspirate pH of 2.5 or less.

Shortly after arrival in the PACU, auscultation of the lungs revealed some end-expiratory wheezes, which responded to nebulized albuterol. As no particulate matter was noted in the vomitus or the material suctioned from the airway and the chest x-ray did not show an area of hypoventilation, bronchoscopy was not indicated. No additional antibiotics were indicated, as these have not proven to be of benefit unless positive cultures are obtained. Steroids are not administered, as they also are of no proven benefit.

The patient was admitted to the intensive care unit (ICU) for overnight observation and repeated nebulized albuterol treatments. Remarkably, he remained stable and was transferred to the unit the next morning without apparent adverse effects from his aspiration. He returned to the operating room early the next week for closure of his wound and was discharged from the hospital shortly thereafter.

LEARNING ACTIVITIES

- ◆ Review your facility's patient assessment data requirements and the routine monitoring requirements, and familiarize yourself with normal and abnormal results.
- ◆ Review institutional policy and procedures for documenting and reporting patient data.
- ◆ Review the *Perioperative Nursing Data Set.*
- ◆ Become certified in basic life support or advanced cardiac life support.
- ◆ Seek out continuing education on physical assessment.
- ◆ Consult perioperative resource books for information regarding how the surgical experience can affect patient data.
- ◆ Become familiar with how age, health, common disease processes, and medications can alter patient data.
- ◆ Create a "cheat sheet" of common patient data parameters to carry with you when caring for patients.
- ◆ If you discover that you are particularly weak in

knowledge of certain areas of patient assessment, seek out continuing education classes in those areas.

RECOMMENDED STUDY MATERIALS

Fortunato, N, ed, *Berry & Kohn's Operating Room Technique*, ninth ed (St Louis: Mosby, Inc, 2000).

Beyea, S, ed, *Perioperative Nursing Data Set.* (Denver: AORN, Inc, 2002).

Meeker, M H; Rothrock, J C, eds, *Alexander's Care of the Patient in Surgery*, 12th ed (St Louis: Mosby, Inc, 2002).

Phippen, M L; Wells, M P, *Patient Care During Operative and Invasive Procedures* (Philadelphia: W B Saunders Co, 2000).

Roth, R A, ed, *Perioperative Nursing Core Curriculum* (Philadelphia: W B Saunders Co, 1995).

Spry, C, *Essentials of Perioperative Nursing*, second ed (Gaithersburg, Md: Aspen Publishers, 1997).

CHAPTER 2: FORMULATE NURSING DIAGNOSES

Nancymarie Fortunato-Phillips, RN, BSN, MEd, CNOR, CPSN

A nursing diagnosis is derived from the nursing assessment data and provides the framework for nursing intervention that enables the patient to attain desired outcomes. It signifies a standardized nursing nomenclature and consists of three parts:

- human response of the patient to health, disease, and the environment—objective signs and subjective symptoms;
- defining characteristics such as a problem, needs, or health status consideration; and
- etiology or related factors supported by medical data.

The differences between the nursing diagnosis and the medical diagnosis are as follows.

- Medical diagnosis: Pathophysiology is determined by the physician after evaluating medical data, laboratory data, x-rays, and other medical processes performed by a physician.
- Nursing diagnosis: Evaluation of human responses to actual or potential problems or conditions by the registered nurse who is responsible for and capable of independent treatment.

The North American Nursing Diagnosis Association (NANDA) has developed an ordered taxonomy of 155 accepted nursing diagnoses that can be used to clearly identify specific diagnoses for each patient. These can be categorized by two methods.

- Human response patterns:
  - exchanging
  - communicating
  - relating
  - valuing
  - choosing
  - moving
  - perceiving
  - knowing
  - fccling
- Functional health patterns:
  - health perception/health management
  - nutritional/metabolic
  - elimination
  - activity/exercise
  - sleep/rest
  - cognitive/perceptual
  - self-perception/self-concept
  - role/relationship
  - sexuality/reproductive
  - coping/stress tolerance
  - value/belief

LEARNING OBJECTIVES

1. Compare and contrast nursing and medical diagnosis processes.
2. Describe the three components of a nursing diagnosis.
3. Analyze and categorize pertinent nursing assessment data into functional health patterns.
4. List four human response patterns assessed by the perioperative nurse in the formulation of a nursing diagnosis.

TASK STATEMENT; AREAS OF KNOWLEDGE AND SKILL

Task Statement

Identify actual or potential clinical problems, needs, or health considerations to direct nursing interventions intended to achieve expected outcomes.

Areas of Knowledge

K-1 Health assessment techniques
K-2 Anatomy and physiology
K-3 Pathophysiology
K-4 Pharmacology and anesthetic agents
K-5 Pain management
K-6 Principles of wound healing
K-7 Diagnostic procedures and results
K-11 Physiologic responses to the surgical experience
K-15 Risks for injury, including but not limited to skin, positioning, and retained foreign body
K-16 Emergency procedures (eg, CPR, MH)
K-17 Postoperative complications
K-18 Defining characteristics of impending patient physiologic crisis
K-20 Sociology (eg, cultural and ethnic influences, family patterns, spirituality and related practices)
K-21 Communication theories and techniques
K-22 Behavioral responses to the surgical experience
K-23 Discharge planning
K-25 *Perioperative Nursing Data Set* (PNDS)
K-27 Microbiology and infection control
K-28 Standard and transmission-based precautions
K-29 Potential hazards in the perioperative environment including but not limited to chemical, electrical, fire, gas, laser, physical environment, radiologic, extraneous objects
K-32 Environmental parameters (eg, temperature, humidity, air exchange)
K-39 Patient rights and responsibilities
K-40 Legal responsibilities and implications for patient care
K-41 Approved nursing diagnoses (eg, NANDA)
K-42 Nursing research and evidence-based practice
K-43 "ANA Code of Ethics for Nurses with Explications for Perioperative Nurses"
K-44 Regulatory standards and voluntary guidelines
K-45 AORN *Standards, Recommended Practices, and Guidelines*
K-46 AORN position statements (eg, bloodborne pathogens, do-not-resuscitate orders [DNR])
K-47 Principles of problem solving
K-48 Quality improvement principles
K-50 Defining characteristics of impaired individuals (eg, substance abuse, psychological disturbance, compromised performance)
K-52 Defining characteristics of domestic abuse (eg, child, elder, partner/spouse)
K-56 Implants (handling, tracking, sterilization)

Areas of Skill

S-1 Confirming patient identity, operative site, and procedure
S-2 Collecting, analyzing, and prioritizing patient data
S-3 Using health assessment techniques (eg, interview, observation, auscultation, palpation, percussion)
S-4 Communicating effectively (verbal and nonverbal)
S-6 Evaluating environment for discharge care
S-7 Assessing and managing pain
S-8 Assessing for potential abuse (eg, substance, domestic)
S-9 Assessing readiness to learn, knowledge level, and preferred learning style
S-10 Identifying barriers to learning
S-11 Identifying risk of infection and injury
S-12 Identifying cultural, spiritual, ethnic issues in care
S-13 Identifying age specific needs
S-14 Formulating a nursing diagnosis
S-15 Collaborating with other members on the health care team
S-16 Applying AORN *Standards, Recommended Practices, and Guidelines*
S-17 Applying the *Perioperative Nursing Data Set* (PNDS)
S-18 Delineating and communicating measurable patient outcomes
S-20 Maintaining accurate patient records
S-22 Providing evidence based care
S-24 Developing a patient and family education plan
S-30 Documenting all relevant facts and data elements with appropriate terminology
S-35 Maintaining the dignity, modesty, and privacy of the patient and protecting the confidentiality of patient information
S-50 Adapting to special and unusual needs
S-54 Recognizing impaired behavior in patients, family, and staff members and responding appropriately
S-60 Directing health care team members in emergency situations
S-61 Performing basic life support and other emergency procedures
S-62 Setting priorities

S-65 Applying ethical principles
S-70 Classifying the surgical wound

PERIOPERATIVE NURSING DIAGNOSIS

The perioperative nursing diagnosis begins with admission of the patient to the presurgical area. The assessment and nursing diagnosis process will be started by the admitting registered nurse. Regardless of the area of the facility beginning the admission, the process will be continued by the perioperative nurse in the operating room suite.

The immediacy of the assessment in the operating suite requires the perioperative nurse to make several nursing diagnoses concurrently.

Example: The patient is lying on the transport cart/bed outside the door to the operating room. The perioperative nurse introduces himself or herself and identifies the patient according to facility policy and procedure. The perioperative nurse reviews the chart for the history and physical, appropriate consents, laboratory reports, and other medical diagnostic data.

In these few moments, several initial parameters such as the following are assessed.

- Human response patterns:
  - exchanging
  - communicating
  - relating
  - perceiving
  - knowing
- Functional health patterns:
  - health perception/management
  - nutritional/metabolic
  - activity/exercise
  - cognitive/perceptual
  - coping/stress tolerance

Data from this initial assessment by the perioperative nurse may identify several nursing diagnoses that may include, but are not limited to,

- knowledge deficit;
- thought processes, altered;
- impaired verbal ability; and
- ineffective coping.

ESTABLISHING THE NURSING DIAGNOSIS

As the patient's identification wristband is checked, the perioperative nurse can use his or her senses of hearing, vision, touch, and smell to expand the assessment. The nurse can visually observe behaviors, skin condition (eg, color, moisture, integrity), and general health. The patient's breath odors can be sensed as he or she answers questions and the answers can be assessed for appropriateness. Nursing diagnoses will stem directly from this interaction. AORN's *Perioperative Nursing Data Set* can be used to establish the common descriptors for stating perioperative nursing diagnoses.

Standardized nursing diagnoses for the intraoperative period may include, but are not limited to, the following.

- Potential for injury related to transport and transfer.
- Potential for injury related to electrical, chemical, radiation, falls, extraneous objects.
- Potential for alterations in body temperature related to hypothermia or hyperthermia.
- Potential for fluid imbalance related to overload or dehydration.
- Potential for alteration in skin integrity related to immobilization, pressure, or shearing forces.
- Potential for pain related to surgical intervention.

SUMMARY

Use of information from the patient's chart in combination with subjective and objective assessment data can be used to formulate the perioperative nursing diagnosis. The plan of care will be built around the nursing diagnoses and should be established on an individual basis. Cultural and ethnic variances should be taken into consideration.

CASE STUDIES

Case Study: Sister CF

Sister CF, age 46, is admitted for abdominal pain and fever. She has no known family other than the Sisters at the Mother House. Several of the Sisters have accompanied her to the hospital. Her vital signs are temperature - 99.8° F, pulse (P) - 102, respiratory rate (RR) - 22, blood pressure (BP) - 130/90. She is very pale and diaphoretic. Her history includes nausea and vomiting of two days duration. She has been NPO for 10 hours. She has an allergy to penicillin that manifests in a rash. Her facial expression is very stoic, and she is lying on her right side with her legs drawn up toward her abdomen. The laboratory technician has drawn her complete blood count, and the results have not yet been called to the presurgical area. Her physician has arranged for a surgical consult with a general surgeon, and the medical plan is to perform an exploratory laparoscopy. Her pending diagnosis is acute appendicitis.

Sister CF has uncorrected scoliosis of the thoracic spine, which prevents her from lying in a supine position. She begins to cry as the perioperative nurse approaches and relates that she is prepared to die if it is her time.

Points to Consider

- The duration of the patient's illness and the state of her hydration may negatively affect her fluid and electrolyte balance.
- The patient may be in a great deal of pain due to an inflamed appendix or due to peritonitis from a ruptured appendix. Pain affects vital signs and the ability of the patient to participate or cooperate in her care.
- CF's scoliosis may prevent the usual positioning for an exploratory laparotomy and may contribute to decreased lung function and possible injury from positioning if not carefully addressed.
- The patient has no family support. She is accompanied by members of her religious order who may offer support, but the philosophy and expectations of this religious order may affect the patient's anxiety levels and her ability to communicate and relate to the perioperative nursing staff and others.
- The patient appears frightened and may have a knowledge deficit regarding her condition and its outcome. She may have a knowledge deficit regarding health and hospitals in general and will need a careful nursing approach, assessment, education, and care to prevent her anxiety from negatively affecting her care and recuperation.

What are some appropriate nursing diagnoses for this patient?

Discussion of Points to Consider

The perioperative nurse can identify the following nursing diagnoses as they apply to this patient.

- Potential for fluid and electrolyte imbalance related to dehydration from vomiting.
- Potential for infection from ruptured appendix.
- Potential for alteration in body temperature related to hyperthermia.
- Potential for pain related to condition and the surgical intervention.
- Potential for anesthesia complications (ie, aspiration on induction) due to disruption in normal gastrointestinal function.
- Potential for injury related to positioning due to presence of scoliosis.
- Potential for alteration in skin integrity related to immobility, pressure, or shear forces.
- Knowledge deficit related to surgical intervention and general health.
- Lack of support system or presence of a dysfunctional support system.
- Potential for ineffective coping.
- Need for psychosocial support and counseling.

Case Study: KW

KW, age 4, is scheduled for release of burn scars on her upper extremities and neck. The child has had several procedures since her initial injury, which occurred in a fire in her foster family's home two months previously. The cause of the fire was a space heater in her bedroom. The social service agency responsible for her care has not sent anyone to be with her for the procedure. Her birth mother placed her in foster care, and her father's whereabouts are unknown.

KW is very restless and crying. She has no interest in her favorite stuffed toy. She is rocking her body back and forth and stiffens her body when touched by any of the staff members. The perioperative nurse notes that when the registered nurse who cared for her in the operating room previously approaches, the child's cries lessen and she tries to say the nurse's name.

Points to Consider

- How does the age and developmental stage of this child affect the nursing approach and care?
- The lack of social support and the trauma of the initial injury and foster care, as well as the failure of social services to provide support for this child makes establishing a relationship difficult but essential.

- The nurse's observation regarding the previous nurse's care and relationship with this child is crucial to providing a positive experience for this child, helping her to cope with her injuries and participate in her care, and preventing negative surgical outcomes.
- Major psychological stages of development may have been thwarted or delayed by the child's perceived abandonment by her primary caregiver (mother) and by the failure of social services and the foster care family to be present, assist with her care, and ease her fears. The child may exhibit regressive behavior during stressful situations (eg, loss of toilet training skills, refusal to speak).
- Because child will probably need multiple surgeries to correct scar tissue and burn sequelae, establishing a positive relationship with at least one member of the nursing staff will be essential for positive outcomes.

What are some appropriate nursing diagnoses for this child in addition to the standard diagnoses required for all pediatric patients?

Discussion of Points to Consider

The child's age and developmental stage as well as the physical and psychological trauma sustained are seen in the following diagnoses.

- Potential for impaired verbal ability.
- Potential for ineffective coping.
- Potential for knowledge deficit.
- Potential for high levels of stress.
- Lack of social support.
- Potential for altered thought processes.
- Need for psychosocial support and counseling.

Case Study: Mr. OP

Mr. OP, age unknown, was brought to the presurgical holding area from the emergency department after a motor vehicle accident. His medical history is unknown, though he is a known street dweller in the neighborhood. His injuries include a fractured femur, several fractured ribs, and multiple abrasions. As the perioperative nurse approaches, she notes the scent of alcohol on his breath and slightly jaundiced sclera, bilaterally. As she touches his wrist to look at the wrist-band, she notes that he is cool and clammy to the touch. Mr. OP opens his eyes as the nurse speaks to him, but she notes that his pupils have become unequal, a distinct change from her initial assessment. He has been breathing regularly, but has now started coughing a grey, purulent mucous.

Points to Consider

- The patient's care may be negatively affected by possible alcohol consumption, probable full stomach, poor liver function, unknown medical history, possible chronic malnutrition, probable respiratory infection, and the possibility of hepatitis or other infectious conditions.
- The patient may be unable or unwilling to cooperate due to alcohol ingestion, possible head injury related to motor vehicle accident, and possibility of shock.
- The patient's change in vital signs and pupil inequality need to be further assessed and brought to the immediate attention of the surgeon and anesthesia care provider.

Discussion of Points to Consider

In addition to the nursing diagnoses that apply to all perioperative patients, the nurse is aware that the following diagnoses pertain to this patient.

- Increased risk for infection—Mr. OP is at increased risk because of his trauma and existing respiratory infection. As a "street dweller," his nutritional status is probably poor and is influenced by his alcohol intake. This will contribute to his difficulty in fighting infection. OP is also at increased risk of transmitting infection. The cause of his "gray, purulent" sputum is unknown as is the cause of his yellow sclera, which may indicate liver dysfunction or infection.
- Risk for ineffective airway clearance and aspiration—Mr. OP is showing signs of deteriorating neurological status because of the change in pupil size, he appears to have ingested alcohol which will negatively affect his reflexes, and he is cool and clammy to the touch and may be experiencing shock. At present he is coughing and appears able to maintain his airway, but this could change if his vital signs deteriorate further. These assessments need to be brought to the attention of the surgeon and anesthesia care provider as soon as possible, and the nurse should ask other preoperative personnel to gather emergency measures for maintaining the patient's airway, while he or she remains with the patient.
- Risk for decreased cardiac output—If Mr. OP has sustained internal injuries, his cool clammy skin may be an early indicator of blood loss and shock. The nurse should be aware that the patient's vital signs need to be monitored closely and fluid replacement/blood products made

available as soon as possible. OP is also at risk for fluid volume and electrolyte imbalance. OP's probable poor nutrition, possible blood loss from the trauma, and suspected internal injuries will all contribute to his fluid and electrolyte imbalance.

- Potential for pain related to condition and the surgical intervention.
- Knowledge deficit related to surgical intervention and general health.

SUGGESTED LEARNING ACTIVITIES

- Practice making lists of nursing diagnoses based on family members. Be certain to assess both adults and children because the problems, needs, and health considerations are widely different. Consider the expected developmental stage, physical parameters, and safety needs.

- Recall a patient in your care from your early years in nursing classes. Try to determine nursing diagnoses that were overlooked by inexperience before you were in practice. List all the things for which you could have provided nursing interventions, such as positioning, safety, and psychological support.

- Take a stroll through the mall and find a comfortable seat. Observe people around you in an unobtrusive way. Notice how many nursing diagnoses are clearly observed in complete strangers. Things to looks for include posture, gait, respiratory effort, and facial signs of stress. Note how they sit and rise from a seated position.

RECOMMENDED STUDY MATERIALS

AORN, *Standards, Recommended Practices, and Guidelines* (Denver: AORN, Inc, 2002).

Beyea, S, ed. *Perioperative Nursing Data Set,* second ed (Denver: AORN Inc, 2002).

Conner, R, ed, *Ambulatory Surgery Principles & Practices*, second ed (Denver: AORN, Inc, 2002).

Fortunato, N, ed, *Berry & Kohn's Operating Room Technique,* ninth ed (St Louis: Mosby, Inc, 2000).

Meeker, M H; Rothrock, J C, eds, *Alexander's Care of the Patient in Surgery,* 12th ed (St Louis: Mosby, Inc, 2002).

North American Nursing Diagnosis Association (NANDA) website: www.nanda.org.

CHAPTER 3: IDENTIFY EXPECTED OUTCOMES

Carol A. Sparks, RN, BSN, CNOR

The perioperative nurse uses the basic nursing process to develop a plan of care. This includes assessment, planning, intervention, and evaluation. As part of the intervention process, the nurse converts a nursing diagnosis into an expected outcome. The 2002 recommended practices and standards of care state that "Patient outcomes are observable, measurable physiologic and psychosocial responses to perioperative nursing interventions."[1] The outcomes reflect the nurse's scope of responsibility in all phases of the perioperative period and are guided by ethical, legal, and moral principles.[2] Outcomes also should reflect age-specific and cultural considerations of the patient population.

Expected outcomes also provide a process by which care can be measured either by verbal questioning of the patient and/or family or by chart review. Outcomes also can provide the framework by which accountability of the efficiency and effectiveness of care can be documented for regulatory or accrediting agencies (eg, Joint Commission on the Accreditation of Healthcare Organizations [JCAHO]).[3]

This chapter provides the perioperative nurse with information related to expected outcomes. The nurse will be able to identify the correlation between defining a nursing diagnosis, developing a plan of care, and defining expected outcomes.

LEARNING OBJECTIVES

When this chapter is completed, the nurse will be able to:

1. Explain the relationship between nursing diagnoses, nursing interventions, and expected patient outcomes.
2. Outline the process for writing an expected patient outcome statement.
3. Describe the process for evaluation of the expected outcome.

TASK STATEMENT; AREAS OF KNOWLEDGE AND SKILL

Task Statement

Identify expected outcomes by using the patient assessment and nursing diagnoses to formulate an individualized age-specific plan of care.

Areas of Knowledge

- K-1 Health assessment techniques
- K-2 Anatomy and physiology
- K-3 Pathophysiology
- K-4 Pharmacology and anesthetic agents
- K-5 Pain management
- K-6 Principles of wound healing
- K-7 Diagnostic procedures and results
- K-9 Surgical, anesthetic, and other perioperative interventions
- K-10 Expected outcomes related to identified interventions
- K-11 Physiologic responses to the surgical experience
- K-12 Principles of positioning
- K-15 Risks for injury, including but not limited to skin, positioning, retained foreign body
- K-16 Emergency procedures (eg, CPR, MH)
- K-17 Postoperative complications
- K-20 Sociology (eg, cultural and ethnic influences, family patterns, spirituality and related practices)
- K-22 Behavioral responses to the surgical experience
- K-23 Discharge planning
- K-25 *Perioperative Nursing Data Set* (PNDS)
- K-27 Microbiology and infection control

K-28 Standard and transmission-based precautions
K-29 Potential hazards in the perioperative environment including, but not limited to, chemical, electrical, fire, gas, laser, physical environment, radiologic, extraneous objects
K-30 Interventions to optimize safety
K-32 Environmental parameters (eg, temperature, humidity, air exchange)
K-39 Patient rights and responsibilities
K-41 Approved nursing diagnoses (eg, NANDA)
K-43 "ANA Code of Ethics for Nurses with Explications for Perioperative Nurses"
K-44 Regulatory standards and voluntary guidelines
K-45 AORN *Standards, Recommended Practices, and Guidelines*
K-46 AORN position statements (eg, bloodborne pathogens, do-not-resuscitate orders [DNR])
K-47 Principles of problem solving
K-48 Quality improvement principles
K-52 Defining characteristics of domestic abuse (eg, child, elder, partner/spouse)
K-56 Implants (handling, tracking, sterilization)

Areas of Skill

S-1 Confirming patient identity, operative site, and procedure
S-2 Collecting, analyzing, and prioritizing patient data
S-3 Using health assessment techniques (eg, interview, observation, auscultation, palpation, percussion)
S-4 Communicating effectively (verbal and nonverbal)
S-5 Advocating and protecting patient rights
S-6 Evaluating environment for discharge care
S-7 Assessing and managing pain
S-8 Assessing for potential abuse (eg, substance, domestic)
S-9 Assessing readiness to learn, knowledge level, and preferred learning style
S-10 Identifying barriers to learning
S-11 Identifying risk of infection and injury
S-12 Identifying cultural, spiritual, ethnic issues in care
S-13 Identifying age specific needs
S-14 Formulating a nursing diagnosis
S-15 Collaborating with other members on the health care team
S-16 Applying AORN *Standards, Recommended Practices, and Guidelines*
S-17 Applying the *Perioperative Nursing Data Set* (PNDS)
S-18 Delineating and communicating measurable patient outcomes
S-20 Maintaining accurate patient records
S-21 Protecting patients and members of the health care team from hazardous conditions
S-22 Providing evidence based care
S-23 Applying regulatory standards and voluntary guidelines
S-24 Developing a patient and family education plan
S-26 Incorporating community and institutional resources into plan of care
S-28 Adapting to changing situations and technologies
S-30 Documenting all relevant facts and data elements with appropriate terminology
S-33 Anticipating the needs for equipment, supplies, and personnel
S-35 Maintaining the dignity, modesty, and privacy of the patient and protecting the confidentiality of patient information
S-40 Preparing the surgical site
S-41 Selecting appropriate protective barrier materials
S-43 Controlling environmental noise
S-46 Anticipating and evaluating the effects of pharmacological and anesthetic agents
S-50 Adapting to special and unusual needs
S-56 Measuring, evaluating, and documenting patient outcomes
S-61 Performing basic life support and other emergency procedures
S-62 Setting priorities
S-65 Applying ethical principles
S-67 Evaluating for signs and symptoms of injury
S-69 Recording devices implanted or explanted during procedures
S-70 Classifying the surgical wound

PREOPERATIVE NURSING ACTIVITIES

The perioperative nurse is involved in all three facets of the continuum of care of the surgical patient. The nurse collaborates with many members of the health care team to formulate a plan of care and define expected outcomes. Some sources from which the perioperative nurse will collect data are the

- patient;
- family member or other support person;
- patient record;
- surgeon, anesthesia care provider, nurse or admitting unit or case manager; and
- care path or clinical path.

The perioperative nurse makes an assessment of the patient and interprets that data to formulate a plan of care. That information includes, but is not limited to,

- history and physical, including past surgeries and the patient's response both physically and psychologically;
- lab and diagnostic data when applicable; and
- any allergies, cultural or age-specific differences, or learning deficits.

An example of the process of defining nursing diagnoses and expected outcomes in the preoperative period follows.

Nursing Diagnosis: Acute pain secondary to surgical procedure.

Expected Outcome: Change the nursing diagnosis (ie, pain) into a measurable response—"The patient demonstrates knowledge of pain management."

Outcome Definition: Patient/family members communicate knowledge of pain management as evidenced by an understanding of the plan for pain assessment and management, including knowledge of pharmacologic and nonpharmacologic interventions.[4]

Outcome Indicators:

- Cognition: Repeats instructions correctly, asks appropriate questions. States dose, purpose, frequency, route, and side effects. Is able to use either analog or pictorial pain scale.
- Affective response: Verbalizes understanding of medication administration and agrees to notify health care provider of inadequate pain relief.
- Psychomotor skills: Is able to demonstrate ability to use patient controlled analgesic (PCA) device or self-administer medications at home.
- Patient satisfaction: Verbalizes satisfaction with pain management teaching.[5]

Nursing Interventions:

- Reviews and validates medication orders.
- Reviews any allergies or sensitivity reactions.
- Evaluates language/cultural/age factors/presence of learning deficits.
- Offers appropriate pain assessment tool (eg, analog or pictorial scale).
- Identifies dose, route, and times of administration.
- Instructs patient/family member on PCA or home administration of medication.
- Reviews desired effects and side effects.
- Encourages notification of health care provider when pain is relieved or worsening.
- Gives instruction on nonpharmacologic pain relief strategies (eg, relaxation, elevation, cold therapy).
- Evaluates verbal and nonverbal response to medication.[6]

INTRAOPERATIVE NURSING ACTIVITIES

There are many nursing diagnoses and expected outcomes in the intraoperative phase of the patient's surgical experience. One example is related to use of electrosurgical unit (ESU).

Nursing Diagnosis: Risk of injury.

Expected Outcome: Change the problem (ie, risk of injury) into a measurable outcome—"The patient is free from signs and symptoms of electrical injury."

Outcome Definition: The patient is free from any observable signs or reported symptoms of injury related to use of ESU.

Outcome Indicators:

- Skin condition: Dispersive electrode site is smooth and intact; free from blisters, redness, ecchymosis.
- Neuromuscular status: Flexes and extends extremities; no numbness or tingling.
- Pain perception: Denies acute pain or discomfort at dispersive electrode side.[7]

Nursing Interventions: Prevents injury secondary to dispersive electrode placement, active electrode, electrosurgical unit, and stray radio frequency current.

- Prevents use in the presence of flammable gases or liquids.
- Limits use in enriched oxygen atmospheres.
- Prevents use in presence of flammable prep agents.
- Prevents pooling of prepping solutions.
- Checks ESU and dispersive electrode for any compromises (eg, frayed wires, packaging not intact).
- Uses dispersive electrode according to manufacturer's guidelines.
- Shaves and cleans application site if necessary.
- Uses appropriate dispersive electrode pad for size and weight of patient (eg, neonate, child, adult).
- Places dispersive electrode in close proximity to the operative site when possible.
- Avoids bony prominences, scar tissue, or metal prosthesis.
- Places active electrode in nonconductive holder when not in use.
- Prevents active electrode from being activated near flammable materials such as patient drapes.
- Sets the generator activation tone at an audible level.
- Checks both the active and the patient dispersive electrode and connections before increasing power settings.
- Cleans eschar buildup from active electrode.
- Avoids excessive coiling or clamping of electrode cords with metal instrument.
- Records placement of dispersive electrode, identification number of unit, and settings used.
- Evaluates and documents integrity at dispersive electrode site, under electrocardiogram (ECG) leads, bony prominences, and/or pressure points at end of procedure.[8]

POSTOPERATIVE NURSING ACTIVITIES

Most expected outcomes are evaluated in the postoperative period. When the actual patient response is similar to the expected outcome, a positive patient outcome is the result. If the outcome is different than that of the expected result, the nurse needs to determine whether the patient has had an adverse event requiring some kind of intervention and then intervene on the patient's behalf. A risk identification report must be filed with the hospital risk management office. If the adverse event is extremely serious, it may be a US Food and Drug Administration (FDA) reportable event.

An example of an expected postoperative outcome follows.

Nursing Diagnosis: Potential for hypothermia.

Expected Outcome: The patient is at or returning to normothermia at the conclusion of immediate postoperative period.

Outcome Indicators:

- Vital signs: Temperature, pulse, and respirations within expected ranges.
- Cardiovascular status: Heart rate and blood pressure within normal ranges. Capillary refill normal.
- Skin condition: Skin warm to touch. Free from shivering, cyanosis, or pallor.[9]

Nursing Interventions: The patient must be near normal temperature for basal metabolic processes to occur. Alterations in temperature, either above or below normothermia, interfere with recovery from anesthesia, increasing the probability of adverse postoperative sequelae. The perioperative nurse must assess those at risk for hypothermia, such as neonates or infants who are at risk because of high body surface/kg and a low subcutaneous tissue reserve. The elderly also are at risk because of low basal metabolic rate, limited cardiovascular reserves, thinning of skin, and reduced muscle mass. Others at risk for hypothermia are patients with traumatic destruction of skin, or those with large exposed wounds for a prolonged period of time.[10]

Interventions include the following.

- Selection of temperature monitoring devices to cool or warm the patient as indicated.

- Use of those devices according to manufacturer's guidelines.
- Monitors and documents patient's pulse, oxygenation saturation (SaO_2), core temperature, respirations, and blood pressure.
- Monitors patient for intraoperative bleeding.
- Listens for patient's verbalization of thermal comfort; notes any shivering.
- Reports to PACU nurse any thermoregulation strategies used and patient response.[11]

Evaluation:

- Verbal and nonverbal information from patient.
- Core temperature and other vital signs.
- Monitors patient for immediate postoperative bleeding.
- Monitors patient for any cardiac dysrhythmia.[12]

SUMMARY

The successful perioperative nurse must use a wide variety of assessment tools to formulate a plan of care for the surgical patient. Based on that assessment, nursing diagnoses are formulated and then expected outcomes are identified. The development and evaluation of patient outcomes is ongoing throughout the surgical experience.

CASE STUDIES

Case Study: Baby A

Baby A is born at 36 weeks gestation via cesarean section secondary to a myelomeningocele. She is coming to the operating room urgently for possible primary closure of a large myelomeningocele.

Nursing assessment reveals that Baby A is a 5-lb. infant who arrives in the OR via transport isolette accompanied by her father, grandmother, and a neonatal intensive care nurse. Her mother is still recovering from the cesarean section. The father is anxious but is being appropriately supported by the grandmother. He is asking appropriate questions. Baby A is intubated, has a SaO_2 of 94% on 30% oxygen, and has an umbilical line in place. Her color is pink, and she is grimacing around the endotracheal tube. She is moving her upper extremities well but has decreased movement in her lower extremities. She has a sterile dressing covering the wound on her back.

Points to Consider

1. What nursing diagnoses are appropriate for Baby A and her family?
2. What are some expected outcomes for Baby A?
3. What outcome indicators would help define the expected outcomes?
4. Think of some nursing interventions appropriate to Baby A.
5. How can you evaluate effectiveness of the care for Baby A?

Discussion of Points to Consider

1. Several nursing diagnoses that are appropriate for Baby A and her family are
    - anxiety related to Baby A's immediate surgical care and potential long-term health concerns;
    - potential for knowledge deficit of Baby A's parents;
    - potential for hypothermia;
    - risk of developing latex allergy; and
    - risk of infection.
2. Some expected outcome definitions for Baby A might be
    - the patient's family exhibits effective coping mechanisms;
    - the patient's family demonstrates knowledge of surgical procedure, baby's prognosis, and future care;
    - baby is normothermic at end of surgical procedure;
    - latex allergy risk is reduced; and
    - the patient is free from signs and symptoms of infection.
3. Some potential outcome indicators related to nursing interventions follow.

    Anxiety and knowledge deficit of parents:
    - Cognition: Family repeats information correctly; asks appropriate questions based on information provided.

- Affective responses: Anxious, but calm and appropriate. Cooperates with plan of care; verbalizes family support and ability to cope.
- Supportive resources: Family demonstrates willingness to participate in long-term care and rehabilitation.
- Patient satisfaction: Family verbalizes satisfaction with health teaching.

Examples of outcome indicators for risk of hypothermia:

- Vital signs: Temperature, pulse, and respirations within expected range.
- Cardiovascular status: Heart rate, blood pressure, and SaO_2 within expected ranges; good capillary refill.
- Skin warm to touch; free from cyanosis.

Examples of outcome indicators for risk of latex allergy:

- There are no outcome indicators for latex allergy at this early stage. It is important to know that Baby A is at high risk for developing a latex allergy because of her neural tube deformity and the need for surgery at such an early age.

Examples of outcome indicators for risk infection:

- Skin condition: Open wound increases chance of infection. Strict asepsis must be maintained throughout the perioperative process.
- Medication regimen: Preoperative antibiotics given according to recommended guidelines.
- Documentation: Wound class and infection control interventions documented according to hospital policy.[13]

4. Nursing Interventions for Baby A related to anxiety and knowledge deficit:
    - Take time to spend with family to give explanations and offer supportive listening.
    - Allow family to verbalize fears.
    - Provide privacy for family to bond with baby before entrance into operating room suite.

    Examples of nursing interventions related to potential for hypothermia follow.

    - Increase room temperature adequately.
    - Leave baby in warming isolette until everyone is ready for transport to OR bed.
    - Cover baby's head to prevent excessive heat loss.
    - Use warming lights or other warming devices according to manufacturer's guidelines.
    - Keep transport isolette plugged in and warming for return trip to neonatal unit.
    - Monitor baby's core temp, vital signs, and SaO_2 during procedure.

    Examples of nursing interventions related to latex allergy:

    - It is important to maintain a latex free environment for baby to decrease risk of latex sensitization and subsequent allergy. Parental teaching of increased risk of latex allergy important and must be followed up.

    Examples of nursing interventions related to infection risk:

    - Performs skin preparation.
    - Maintains sterile environment and monitors aseptic technique throughout entire surgical experience.
    - Administers medications according to established guidelines.
    - Places sterile dressing on.

5. Examples to demonstrate evaluation and effectiveness of interventions and expected outcomes:
    - Family verbalizes appropriate communication and coping mechanisms.
    - Baby is normothermic at completion of surgical procedure.
    - A latex free environment has been maintained and documented.
    - Wounds and other invasive sites are covered in sterile dressings.
    - Wound classification documented.

Summary

This case study listed just a few examples of nursing diagnoses, interventions, and expected outcomes for Baby A. The perioperative nurse must constantly assess the patient's changing condition to determine what expected outcomes are met, must be changed, or added to the plan of care.

Case Study: Ms. T

Ms. T is a 29-year-old woman who is being admitted for an elective arthroscopic anterior cruciate ligament (ACL) repair for an injury sustained while skiing. Other than her knee injury, she is in excellent physical health and does not smoke. She reports to the ambulatory care center with her husband. The patient has a knee immobilizer on and is ambulating on crutches. When asked about her pain, she reports that one half hour after taking two Percocets (oxycodone HCl and acetaminophen), her pain is still 3 to 4 on a 1-10 scale. She reports no allergies and will be having an epidural anesthetic. She has not had surgery in the past.

Points to Consider

1. What are some of the nursing diagnoses that will govern your care of Ms. T?

2. What are some of the nursing interventions that will be used?

3. What are some of the expected outcomes of Ms. T's surgical experience?

4. How can you elevate those expected outcomes?

Discussion of Points to Consider

1. What are some of the nursing diagnoses that will govern your care of Ms. T?
   - Patient is experiencing acute pain and will continue to experience acute pain in the postoperative period.
   - Patient is at risk of injury secondary to devices that will be used during surgery, such as the tourniquet and ESU.
   - Patient is at risk for impaired mobility.

2. What are some of the nursing interventions that will be used?
   - Assess patient's pain in the preoperative, intraoperative, and postoperative periods. Review medication regimen protocol and other pain reduction strategies, such as extremity elevation and ice application. Encourage family participation in pain management.
   - Interventions to ensure safe use of ESU and peripheral tourniquet. Examines equipment for proper functioning and safety before patient enters the room. Places the dispersive electrode and tourniquet according to manufacturer's recommendations. Maintains skin integrity and monitors according to hospital policy.
   - Patient is instructed in proper crutch walking and importance of maintaining mobility.

3. What are some of the expected outcomes of Ms. T's surgical experience?
   - Patient will demonstrate knowledge of pain management and be able to effectively manage pain.
   - Patient will be free from injury related to tourniquet and ESU use.
   - Patient will maintain mobility and demonstrate safe crutch walking.

4. How can you elevate those expected outcomes?
   - Frequently assessing patient's pain using analog scale. Getting verbal and nonverbal confirmation from patient regarding pain relief. Following up with patient by telephone call on the first postoperative day and by giving patient advice on what to do if pain relief is not adequate.
   - Maintains record of ESU and tourniquet use including informing surgeon of tourniquet time at established intervals. At end of procedure, inspects skin at dispersive electrode and tourniquet sites for any bruising or blistering. Checks peripheral pulses and capillary refill at end of procedure.
   - Reports postoperative interventions and findings to PACU nurse for further evaluation.
   - Patient and family verbalize importance of early and frequent mobilization. Demonstrates safe crutch walking.

Summary

The experienced perioperative nurse will have gathered the necessary knowledge to critically assess the patient; formulate nursing diagnoses, a plan of care, and expected outcomes; and effectively evaluate that care. Perioperative patients have many similar and unique facets of their experience and the perioperative nurse must be able to constantly re-evaluate and adjust care accordingly.

SUGGESTED LEARNING ACTIVITIES

◆ Review AORN's *Standard, Recommended Practices, and Guidelines* and the *Perioperative Nursing Data Set.*

◆ Review your institution's policies and procedures regarding nursing care plans and the documentation of nursing diagnoses, interventions, and outcomes.

◆ Practice making nursing care plans and reviewing your current nursing care plans to evaluate your strengths and weaknesses. In what areas do you need the most practice?

- Review perioperative nursing texts (eg, *Alexander's Care of the Patient in Surgery, Berry & Kohn's Operating Room Technique, Care of the Patient During Operative and Invasive Procedures*) for further information regarding formulating nursing care plans.
- Consult with peers regarding nursing care plans and how you could improve.

REFERENCES

1. AORN, *Standards, Recommended Practices, and Guidelines* (Denver: AORN, 2002) 17.
2. S Beyea, ed, *Perioperative Nursing Data Set* (Denver: AORN, 2002) 21.
3. N Fortunato, ed, *Berry & Kohn's, Operating Room Technique* ninth ed (St Louis: Mosby, Inc, 2000).
4. *Perioperative Nursing Data Set,* 139.
5. *Ibid.*
6. *Ibid.*
7. *Ibid*, 94.
8. *Ibid.*
9. *Ibid,* 121.
10. *Ibid.*
11. *Ibid.*
12. *Ibid.*
13. *Ibid*, 105.

RECOMMENDED STUDY MATERIALS

AORN, *Standards, Recommended Practices, and Guidelines* (Denver: AORN, Inc, 2002).

Beyea, S, ed, *Perioperative Nursing Data Set,* second ed (Denver: AORN, Inc, 2002).

Fairchild, S, *Perioperative Nursing: Principles and Practice,* second ed (Boston: Little, Brown and Company, 1996).

Fortunato, N, ed, *Berry & Kohn's, Operating Room Technique* ninth ed (St Louis: Mosby, Inc, 2000).

Groah, L, *Perioperative Nursing,* third ed (Stamford, Conn: Appleton and Lange, 1996).

Phippen, M L; Wells, M P, *Patient Care During Operative and Invasive Procedures* (Philadelphia: W B Saunders Co, 2000).

Roth, R, ed, *Perioperative Nursing Core Curriculum* (Philadelphia: W B Saunders Co, 1995).

Spry, C, *Essentials of Perioperative Nursing,* second ed (Gaithersburg, Md: Aspen Publishers, 1997).

CHAPTER 4:

DEVELOP PLAN OF CARE

Dru A. Beedle, RN, MN, CNOR, CNA

Perioperative nurses develop a plan of care after patient assessment has been completed, nursing diagnoses have been formulated, and patient care outcomes have been identified. Planning, which is the fourth step in the nursing process, is often referred to as the heart and soul of nursing. Care plan development is the foundation of nursing care and fundamental to our nursing practice. The plan of care will direct all nursing care activities related to each patient.

Developing a plan of care actually begins when a patient is scheduled for surgery and ends when the patient is discharged. In some cases, the planning phase can extend to postoperative telephone calls made by the perioperative nurse or when the perioperative nurse sees the patient on a return postoperative visit. Developing a plan of care is the basic, systematic process of identifying patient outcomes and determining how to achieve them. Simply put, the perioperative nurse must

- decide what needs to be done,
- when it needs to be done,
- how it needs to be done,
- where it needs to be done, and
- who is to do it.

The perioperative nurse develops a plan of care that identifies nursing interventions to meet identified outcomes. Developing a plan of care gives direction, guidance, and meaning to perioperative nursing care. Purposes of plan of care development include

- provide for continuity of patient care,
- identify patient care activities for the nursing care team,
- allow for appropriate delegation to qualified personnel,
- identify the appropriate setting for care delivery,
- individualize care for each patient,
- prioritize care for each patient, and
- provide means to communicate nursing process activities to the health care team.

This chapter addresses the theoretical approach to developing a plan of care for the surgical patient. Specific nursing interventions are identified in this chapter, and the written plan of care is discussed.

LEARNING OBJECTIVES

1. Discuss importance of individualized care plan development.
2. Identify factors to consider when developing a plan of care for perioperative patients.
3. Differentiate nurse initiated and physician prescribed interventions.
4. List the AORN recommended practice nursing interventions that should be incorporated into the surgical patient's plan of care.
5. Compare and contrast a standardized nursing care plan and critical pathway.

TASK STATEMENT; AREAS OF KNOWLEDGE AND SKILL

Task Statement

Develop a plan of care based on assessment of the patient that includes the nursing diagnoses, expected outcomes, and nursing interventions necessary to achieve desired results.

Areas of Knowledge

K-1 Health assessment techniques
K-2 Anatomy and physiology
K-3 Pathophysiology
K-4 Pharmacology and anesthetic agents
K-5 Pain management
K-6 Principles of wound healing
K-7 Diagnostic procedures and results
K-8 Preoperative patient preparation activities
K-9 Surgical, anesthetic, and other perioperative interventions
K-10 Expected outcomes related to identified interventions
K-11 Physiologic responses to the surgical experience
K-12 Principles of positioning
K-14 Transfer and transport techniques and equipment
K-15 Risks for injury, including but not limited to, skin, positioning, and retained foreign body
K-16 Emergency procedures (eg, CPR, MH)
K-17 Postoperative complications
K-18 Defining characteristics of impending patient physiologic crisis
K-20 Sociology (eg, cultural and ethnic influences, family patterns, spirituality and related practices)
K-21 Communication theories and techniques
K-22 Behavioral responses to the surgical experience
K-23 Discharge planning
K-24 Theories of and resources for patient/family education
K-25 *Perioperative Nursing Data Set* (PNDS)
K-26 Requirements for handling of specimens
K-27 Microbiology and infection control
K-28 Standard and transmission-based precautions
K-29 Potential hazards in the perioperative environment including, but not limited to, chemical, electrical, fire, gas, laser, physical environment, radiologic, and extraneous objects
K-30 Interventions to optimize safety
K-31 Technologies and equipment relating to perioperative practice
K-32 Environmental parameters (eg, temperature, humidity, air exchange)
K-39 Patient rights and responsibilities
K-40 Legal responsibilities and implications for patient care
K-41 Approved nursing diagnoses (eg, NANDA)
K-42 Nursing research and evidence-based practice
K-43 "ANA Code of Ethics for Nurses with Explications for Perioperative Nurses"
K-44 Regulatory standards and voluntary guidelines
K-45 AORN *Standards, Recommended Practices, and Guidelines*
K-46 AORN position statements (eg, bloodborne pathogens, do-not-resuscitate orders [DNR])
K-47 Principles of problem solving
K-49 Surgical consent laws and policies
K-50 Defining characteristics of impaired individuals (eg, substance abuse, psychological disturbance, compromised performance)
K-52 Defining characteristics of domestic abuse (eg, child, elder, partner/spouse)
K-53 Rules, responsibilities, and duties of health care team members and internal and external support service personnel
K-54 Organ procurement
K-55 Credentialing standards and clinical privileges
K-56 Implants (eg, handling, tracking, sterilization)

Areas of Skill

S-1 Confirming patient identity, operative site, and procedure
S-2 Collecting, analyzing, and prioritizing patient data
S-3 Using health assessment techniques (eg, interview, observation, auscultation, palpation, percussion)
S-4 Communicating effectively (verbal and nonverbal)
S-5 Advocating and protecting patient rights
S-6 Evaluating environment for discharge care
S-7 Assessing and managing pain
S-8 Assessing for potential abuse (eg, substance, domestic)
S-9 Assessing readiness to learn, knowledge level, and preferred learning style
S-10 Identifying barriers to learning
S-11 Identifying risk of infection and injury
S-12 Identifying cultural, spiritual, ethnic issues in care
S-13 Identifying age specific needs
S-14 Formulating a nursing diagnosis
S-15 Collaborating with other members on the health care team
S-16 Applying AORN *Standards, Recommended Practices, and Guidelines*
S-17 Applying the *Perioperative Nursing Data Set* (PNDS)

S-18 Delineating and communicating measurable patient outcomes
S-20 Maintaining accurate patient records
S-21 Protecting patients and members of the health care team from hazardous conditions
S-22 Providing evidence-based care
S-23 Applying regulatory standards and voluntary guidelines
S-24 Developing a patient and family education plan
S-25 Applying principles of and participate in, cost-containment, product evaluation, and resource management
S-26 Incorporating community and institutional resources into plan of care
S-27 Delegating interventions and/or assigning tasks
S-28 Adapting to changing situations and technologies
S-29 Performing nursing interventions
S-30 Documenting all relevant facts and data elements with appropriate terminology
S-32 Applying principles and techniques of transport, transfer, and positioning
S-33 Anticipating the needs for equipment, supplies, and personnel
S-34 Applying principles and techniques of body mechanics/ergonomics
S-35 Maintaining the dignity, modesty, and privacy of the patient and protecting the confidentiality of patient information
S-36 Applying principles of aseptic technique and infection control
S-37 Applying principles of sterilization and disinfection
S-38 Applying principles of environmental cleaning
S-40 Preparing the surgical site
S-41 Selecting appropriate protective barrier materials
S-42 Conducting biological monitoring
S-43 Controlling environmental noise
S-44 Testing and using equipment
S-45 Monitoring physiological parameters
S-46 Anticipating and evaluating the effects of pharmacological and anesthetic agents
S-48 Detecting significant changes in the environment
S-49 Preparing and handling specimens for diagnostic evaluation
S-50 Adapting to special and unusual needs
S-51 Identifying and communicating changes in patient status
S-53 Educating, mentoring, and supervising health care team members
S-54 Recognizing impaired behavior in patients, family, and staff and responding appropriately
S-55 Recognizing personal limitations and seeking assistance as needed
S-56 Measuring, evaluating, and documenting patient outcomes
S-58 Identifying appropriate packaging materials for sterilization
S-59 Selecting appropriate and cost-effective sterilization methods
S-60 Directing health care team members in emergency situations
S-61 Performing basic life support and other emergency procedures
S-62 Setting priorities
S-65 Applying ethical principles
S-67 Evaluating for signs and symptoms of injury
S-69 Recording devices implanted or explanted during procedures
S-70 Classifying the surgical wound
S-71 Securing patient belongings and valuables

PERIOPERATIVE NURSING ACTIVITIES

Developing the Plan of Care

Patient assessment, formulation of nursing diagnoses, and identification of expected patient outcomes are important steps in the nursing process. Planning perioperative nursing care is the next sequential step in the ongoing nursing process. Perioperative nursing care plans should incorporate

- physical, social, psychological, and spiritual assessment data from patient, family, and/or significant other;
- collaborative findings from family members and other health care team members;
- formulated nursing diagnoses;
- identified achievable patient outcomes;
- theoretical and clinical knowledge;
- *Perioperative Nursing Data Set* (PNDS) standardized language;
- current recommended clinical practices for perioperative nursing;
- institutional and regulatory recommendations, guidelines, and policies; and
- critical thinking.

The plan of care is a critical component of patient care as identified by the Joint Commission for the

Accreditation of Healthcare Organizations. A patient's care plan needs to be collaborative and regularly reviewed to ensure that it is up-to date and reflects the patient's status changes. Perioperative nurses will develop a plan of care in collaboration with the patient, family, and other health care team members.

Care plans need to be prioritized and sequenced. Factors that will influence the priority of the intervention include

- urgency of the problem,
- nature of treatment indicated, and
- interaction among diagnoses.

A nursing diagnosis that could result in harm or injury to the patient if left untreated should have the highest priority. Using Maslow's hierarchy of needs can help the perioperative nurse prioritize the plan of care. Higher priority should be assigned to physiological, safety and security, and love and belonging needs while lower priority can be assigned to self-esteem and self-actualization needs.

Nursing Actions

Nursing knowledge, experience, and judgment, along with critical thinking skills, are needed to establish care priorities. The established outcome statements will become the guide to determining nursing actions.

There are two categories of nursing actions that can be used to develop the plan of care for perioperative patients—nurse initiated and physician prescribed interventions. Nurse initiated interventions are independent nursing interventions, strategies, or actions that perioperative nurses identify to meet desired outcomes. These actions are defined within the nurse practice act of each state, organizational policies, and professional practice guidelines. Perioperative nurses are able to write nursing orders to treat identified nursing diagnoses.

The *Perioperative Nursing Data Set* (PNDS) identifies independent nursing interventions related to nurse sensitive outcomes in the perioperative setting. The PNDS provides a standardized nursing language or vocabulary defining expected outcomes of perioperative patients and perioperative nursing interventions to achieve these outcomes. Most surgical patients will have an outcome statement stating the patient will be free from signs and symptoms of infection. Some examples of nurse initiated nursing interventions that would be identified on the care plan include

- implement aseptic technique,
- perform skin preparation,
- monitor traffic control, and
- assess wound and identify wound classification.

Physician prescribed interventions are the physician's written orders. The perioperative nurse intervenes by carrying out the prescribed order. Preparing patients for surgery, dispensing medication, initiating treatment, and changing dressings are examples of physician initiated interventions. The perioperative nurse will always use nursing knowledge, skills, and judgment before incorporating a physician prescribed intervention into the plan of care.

According to the AORN 2002 *Standards, Recommended Practices, and Guidelines,* the following interventions should be incorporated into the surgical patient's plan of care:

- provision of information and supportive perioperative teaching specifically related to the surgical intervention and nursing care,
- identification of the patient,
- verification of site and side,
- verification of the operative consent and reports of essential diagnostic procedures,
- positioning according to physiological principles,
- adherence to principles of asepsis,
- provision of appropriate and properly functioning equipment and supplies,
- provision for comfort measures and supportive care for the patient,
- environmental monitoring and safety,
- evaluation of outcomes in relation to the identified interventions, and
- communication of intraoperative information to

significant others and the health care team to provide for continuity of care.

Communicating the Plan of Care

Communicating the plan of care is as important as planning the interventions. Clear and concise nursing interventions have to be written and communicated to all members of the care team. There are numerous methods in the perioperative setting to communicate a plan of care. Standardized nursing care plans and critical pathways are two commonly used methods in the perioperative setting. Facilities may use a computerized care plan design, notebook, or file sheets. Currently, computerized care plans are commonly used as a guide or reference tool to develop a plan of care for each patient. Every care plan form must be developed to reflect individualized nursing diagnoses, patient outcomes, and nursing interventions. A surgeon preference card is not a care plan, but a reference tool to be used to assist perioperative nurses in developing a plan of care.

The standardized nursing care plan has usually been written by a group of perioperative nurses who are experts in their given specialty practice. The care plan is written for a specific population of patients undergoing specific surgeries (eg, hysterectomy, total knee replacement, laparoscopic cholecystectomy). Most common nursing diagnoses are labeled, outcome statements are listed, and routine nursing actions are identified. When using a standardized nursing care plan, perioperative nurses must individualize the care to the specific needs assessed for each patient.

A critical pathway or path is a form of collaborative care planning that is frequently used in health care facilities. Management of quality outcomes is the focus of these multi-disciplinary care plans, while management of procedural costs is a secondary focus of many critical pathways. Collaboration is a key factor in the development of a critical pathway. All health care disciplines involved in the care of a specific population of patients participate to develop the integrated care plan. Critical pathways identify nursing diagnoses, desired outcomes, and interventions of the entire health care team along a defined timeline. Critical pathways are written so that all members of the care team can document interventions, changes in status, or variation from the established plan of care. Variations in all components of the pathway can easily be obtained, analyzed, and trended.

Despite the differences in forms, every plan of care needs to incorporate nursing diagnoses, expected outcomes, and nursing interventions. Individualizing the care to each specific patient is paramount to the successful attainment of quality patient outcomes.

Modifying the Plan of Care

Developing a plan of care is a process that does not end when the care plan has been written or agreed upon. The plan of care must now be implemented and modified as the patient's status changes. Adjusting the plan and modifying the care plan is a key factor to successful and positive patient outcomes.

Developing a plan of care for the perioperative patient is an on-going process. Any change in assessment data, patient needs, or surgical procedure will require the perioperative nurse to potentially modify or change a nursing diagnosis and expected patient outcome. These changes may result in additional or revised nursing interventions. Evaluation and reassessment are subsequent steps in the nursing process that help perioperative nurses meet the needs of each patient and improve upon the planning process for the next patient.

SUMMARY

Care plan development is the foundation of nursing care and fundamental to our nursing practice. The plan of care is the fourth step in the nursing process following assessment, nursing diagnoses identification, and patient outcome identification. Planning and providing patient care must be individualized, responsive, and appropriate to the patients ever changing needs and delivered by qualified perioperative personnel. Professional nursing knowledge, judgment, and critical thinking skills are necessary for the development of a quality, individualized plan of care for perioperative patients.

CASE STUDY

Case Study: Mrs. B

You arrive at work on Monday morning and see that you are scheduled as the circulating nurse for Room 1. The first patient, 43-year-old Mrs. B is scheduled for a laparoscopic cholecystectomy. The patient has just arrived in the surgical admission area. During the course of admission the perioperative nurse notes that the patient is 5'5" and 285 pounds. Her blood pressure is 150/100 with a pulse of 80 and a temperature of 98.9° F. She is allergic to iodine. Mrs. B is a married mother of two with her last son going off to college next week. She is a Jehovah's Witness and has signed documentation stating that she wishes to receive no blood or blood products. All laboratory and diagnostic testing is within normal, but you are unable to find the results of her pregnancy test. Mrs. B's medical history includes a diagnosis of asthma which is controlled by an inhaler and hypertension controlled by medication. Past medical history includes an appendectomy 25 years ago, two C-sections, and a knee arthroscopy. She presents with a cast on her right arm from a fracture secondary to a motor vehicle accident four weeks ago.

Points to Consider

- Where do you begin in the planning of this patient's care?
- Do you have a standardized care plan or critical pathway established to use as a guide to list nursing diagnoses, identify expected patient outcomes, and establish nursing interventions?
- How will you modify your institutional nursing care plan to address the specific needs of Mrs. B?
- Which needs do you consider a priority?
- What resources do you need to have available (eg, personnel, supplies, equipment)?
- What are the individual positioning considerations?
- What teaching will you provide?
- How will you communicate your plan of care to other health care team members?

Discussion of Points to Consider

- Your institutional care plan should be reviewed to help you formulate an appropriate care plan for this patient.

- It is always important to note what patient conditions or complicating factors will cause you to modify your institution's routine nursing care plan. The following patient conditions are a priority and will need special attention in your individualized nursing care plan.
  Obesity: This may present transfer, positioning, and skin care problems. Mrs. B's obesity may have contributed to the previous knee arthroscopy, and she must be assessed for range of motion restrictions.
  Hypertension: Mrs. B's hypertension does not appear well controlled. This will affect tissue perfusion and may increase her tendency to bleed both during and after surgery.
  Allergies: Iodine allergy can be a problem and require the use of alternate scrub/prep solutions. It also may prohibit the use of iodine-based radiographic contrast material if an intraoperative cholangiogram is needed.
  Religious beliefs: These prohibit the use of blood or blood products in a patient who could have bleeding problems.
  Respiratory status: The patient's asthma will affect her respiratory response to stress, anesthesia, and pain.
  Current injury: Mrs. B's arm fracture will present positioning concerns and mobility and protection needs must be assessed.

- You will need help transferring and positioning this patient. In all probability you will need extra personnel to help with the transfer, positioning aids once the patient is on the bed, and possible bed extensions or oversized arm boards, restraints, padding, and protection. The patient will probably need antiembolic stockings or pneumatic compression devices to prevent blood pooling in her extremities during the procedure. This patient will need to be positioned with care, and it will be helpful if she can assist with positioning before induction. Pressure points need to be padded and extremities moved with care so as not to inflict positioning injuries. Pooling of prep solutions is a consideration in patients who are obese. Skin folds should be inspected and dried to prevent chemical injury from prolonged contact with these solutions.

- Depending on the situation and the receptivity of the patient, teaching about weight loss and exercise in the management of hypertension may be helpful. Postoperative breathing regimens and exercise instruction can help this patient recover more quickly. Teaching about signs and symptoms of infection and expected postoperative comfort levels are helpful, and the patient should be instructed on what to report to her surgeon.

- A review of the patient's previous surgical charts (if possible) may be helpful in anticipating and preventing problems. Communication with the anesthesia care provider, the surgeon, and other perioperative personnel is essential. Plans will need to be made for providing medication to control the patient's hypertension and asthma and for replacing any blood loss with alternatives to blood or blood products. Positioning can be discussed and planned for. Alternatives to iodine can be discussed and provided. The radiology department personnel can be consulted and alerted to the patient's iodine allergy and the possible need for intraoperative cholangiograms.

SUGGESTED LEARNING ACTIVITIES

- Discuss perioperative care plan development with your peers.
- Discuss your priorities and rationalizations for your diagnoses, interventions, and outcomes.
- Provide examples for similar experiences with patients, the plan you developed, and the evaluation of the care provided based on assessment, diagnosis, outcomes, and interventions.
- Review AORN's *Standards, Recommended Practices, and Guidelines* and the *Perioperative Nursing Data Set.*
- Review your institution's policies and procedures regarding nursing care plans and the documentation of nursing diagnoses, interventions, and outcomes.
- Review perioperative nursing texts (eg, *Alexander's Care of the Patient in Surgery, Berry & Kohn's Operating Room Technique, Care of the Patient During Operative and Invasive Procedures*) for further information regarding formulating nursing care plans.

RECOMMENDED STUDY MATERIALS

AORN, *Standards, Recommended Practices, and Guidelines* (Denver: AORN, Inc, 2002).

Beyea, S C, "Data fields for intraoperative records using the Perioperative Nursing Data Set," *AORN Journal* 73 (May 2001) 952-954.

Beyea, S, ed, *Perioperative Nursing Data Set*, second ed (Denver: AORN, Inc, 2002).

Carpenito, L J, *Handbook of Nursing Diagnosis,* eighth ed (Philadelphia: J B Lippincott, 1999).

Craven, R F; Hirnle, C J, *Fundamentals of Nursing Human Health and Function,* second ed (Philadelphia: J B Lippincott, 1996).

Fortunato, N H, *Berry & Kohn's Operating Room Technique*, ninth ed (St Louis: Mosby, Inc, 2000).

Joint Commission on Accreditation of Healthcare Organizations, *2002 Hospital Accreditation Standards: Accreditation Policies, Standards, Intent Statements* (Oakbrook, Ill: Joint Commission on Accreditation of Healthcare Organizations, 2002).

Meeker, M H; Rothrock, J D, eds, *Alexander's Care of the Patient in Surgery*, 12th ed (St Louis: Mosby, Inc, 2002).

Potter, P A; Perry, A G, *Fundamentals of Nursing*, fifth ed (St Louis: Mosby, Inc, 2001).

Roth, R A, ed, *Perioperative Nursing Core Curriculum* (Philadelphia: W B Saunders Co, 1995).

Spry, C, *Essentials of Perioperative Nursing* (Gaithersburg, Md: Aspen Publishers, Inc, 1997).

CHAPTER 5: IMPLEMENT PLAN OF CARE TO PREVENT PHYSICAL INJURY

Brenda S. Gregory Dawes, RN, MSN, CNOR

Assessment, planning, and appropriate responses (ie, interventions) to patient needs can prevent physical injury that can occur during an operative or other invasive procedure. Injury can be the result of incorrect use or fault with equipment or supplies or unmet patient care needs.

Patient assessment provides information so that nurses can make judgments concerning patient care management and nursing decisions regarding implementation of patient care before, during, and after the operative or other invasive procedure. Decision making based on critical thinking requires that the nurse respond to a situation or patient care need using knowledge and expertise that will benefit a particular patient. Assessment information enables the perioperative nurse to formulate a plan of care that will achieve anticipated and desirable outcomes. Assessment to achieve the outcome "The patient is free from signs and symtoms of injury" requires an understanding of the patient's physical condition prior to the surgical procedure as well as handling and use of equipment and supplies required to care for the patient. The data is correlated to formulate nursing diagnoses and a plan of care that can be used as a guide for interventions and evaluation.

Within the domain of safety, perioperative nurses should expect that the patient will be free from acquired physical injury. This results in absence of signs and symptoms of physical injury unrelated to the intended therapeutic effects of an operative or other invasive procedure. Injuries can occur during the perioperative period and can result from incorrect use or handling of supplies and equipment, faulty equipment, physiological responses (eg, neuroendocrine responses, metabolic responses), or unmet patient care needs. Preventing injury requires that the nurse understand the patient's systems status including musculoskeletal, neurological, vascular, integumentary, and renal as well as their nutritional status. Understanding their psychological status also is important to prevent physical injury, particularly when the patient will undergo a procedure with moderate or minimal sedation. In addition, the environment (eg, operating room) must be assessed to determine if the functional equipment and protective supplies are available and prepared. Surgeon preferences are identified and modifications in care are made based on patient specific needs. The type of anesthesia planned and expected patient outcomes are identified to provide optimum care through appropriate planning. Thorough assessment enables the nurse to provide individualized patient care that might require modifications of routine practices.

After implementation, the patient is evaluated as special patient care needs are identified and changes in care occur or when the procedure is completed. Interim outcomes are those that can be identified at the point of care and may be indicative of the long-term outcome. For example, an interim outcome might be evaluated at the completion of the operative procedure, but it is necessary to verify the status when the patient is recovered to determine the final outcome status.

LEARNING OBJECTIVES

1. Identify assessment criteria that directly relate to preventing physical injury.
2. Recognize patient care priorities to consider when developing a plan of carc.
3. Discuss nursing interventions that are implemented that prevent physical injury.
4. Demonstrate evaluation skills for those activities implemented to prevent physical injury.

TASK STATEMENT; AREAS OF KNOWLEDGE AND SKILL

Task Statement

Prevent physical injury by providing care that minimizes the risk associated with extraneous objects, chemical injury, electrical injury, transfer/transport, positioning, laser injury, radiation injury, and medication administration.

Areas of Knowledge

K-1 Health assessment techniques
K-2 Anatomy and physiology
K-3 Pathophysiology
K-4 Pharmacology and anesthetic agents
K-5 Pain management
K-6 Principles of wound healing
K-7 Diagnostic procedures and results
K-8 Preoperative patient preparation activities
K-9 Surgical, anesthetic, and other perioperative interventions
K-11 Physiologic responses to the surgical experience
K-12 Principles of positioning
K-13 Ergonomics and body mechanics
K-14 Transfer and transport techniques and equipment
K-15 Risks for injury, including but not limited to, chemical, electrical, fire, gas, laser, physical environment, radiologic, extraneous objects
K-16 Emergency procedures (eg, CPR, MH)
K-20 Sociology (eg, cultural and ethnic influences, family patterns, spirituality and related practices)
K-21 Communication theories and techniques
K-22 Behavioral responses to the surgical experience
K-24 Theories of and resources for patient/family education
K-25 *Perioperative Nursing Data Set* (PNDS)
K-26 Requirements for handling of specimens
K-27 Microbiology and infection control
K-28 Standard and transmission-based precautions
K-29 Potential hazards in the perioperative environment including but not limited to chemical, electrical, fire, gas, laser, physical environment, radiologic, extraneous objects
K-30 Interventions to optimize safety
K-31 Technologies and equipment relating to perioperative practice
K-32 Environmental parameters (eg, temperature, humidity, air exchange)
K-33 Principles of sterilization and disinfection
K-34 Protective barrier materials
K-35 Packaging materials
K-36 Principles of equipment inspection, maintenance, and repair
K-37 Principles of product evaluation, cost-containment, and resource management
K-38 Emergency preparedness (eg, fire, disaster)
K-39 Patient rights and responsibilities
K-40 Legal responsibilities and implications for patient care
K-42 Nursing research and evidence-based practice
K-43 "ANA Code of Ethics for Nurses with Explications for Perioperative Nurses"
K-44 Regulatory standards and voluntary guidelines
K-45 AORN *Standards, Recommended Practices, and Guidelines*
K-46 AORN position statements (eg, bloodborne pathogens, do-not-resuscitate orders [DNR])
K-47 Principles of problem solving
K-49 Surgical consent laws and policies
K-50 Defining characteristics of impaired individuals (eg, substance abuse, psychological disturbance, compromised performance)
K-51 Inappropriate workplace behaviors (eg, harassment, workplace violence)
K-53 Rules, responsibilities, and duties of health care team members and internal and external support service personnel
K-54 Organ procurement
K-55 Credentialing standards and clinical privileges
K-56 Implants (eg, handling, tracking, sterilization)

Areas of Skill

S-1 Confirming patient identity, operative site, and procedure
S-2 Collecting, analyzing, and prioritizing patient data
S-3 Using health assessment techniques (eg, interview, observation, auscultation, palpation, percussion)
S-4 Communicating effectively (verbal and nonverbal)
S-5 Advocating and protecting patient rights
S-6 Evaluating environment for discharge care
S-7 Assessing and managing pain
S-8 Assessing for potential abuse (eg, substance, domestic)
S-9 Assessing readiness to learn, knowledge level, and preferred learning style
S-10 Identifying barriers to learning
S-11 Identifying risk of infection and injury
S-12 Identifying cultural, spiritual, ethnic issues in care
S-13 Identifying age specific needs
S-14 Formulating a nursing diagnosis
S-15 Collaborating with other members on the health care team

S-16 Applying AORN *Standards, Recommended Practices, and Guidelines*
S-17 Applying the *Perioperative Nursing Data Set* (PNDS)
S-18 Delineating and communicating measurable patient outcomes
S-19 Participating in quality improvement activities
S-20 Maintaining accurate patient records
S-21 Protecting patients and members of the health-care team from hazardous conditions
S-22 Providing evidence based care
S-23 Applying regulatory standards and voluntary guidelines
S-24 Developing a patient and family education plan
S-26 Incorporating community and institutional resources into plan of care
S-27 Delegating interventions and/or assigning tasks
S-28 Adapting to changing situations and technologies
S-29 Performing nursing interventions
S-30 Documenting all relevant facts and data elements with appropriate terminology
S-31 Recording unusual occurrences and/or variances in care
S-32 Applying principles and techniques of transport, transfer, and positioning
S-33 Anticipating the needs for equipment, supplies, and personnel
S-34 Applying principles and techniques of body mechanics/ergonomics
S-35 Maintaining the dignity, modesty, and privacy of the patient and protecting the confidentiality of patient information
S-43 Controlling environmental noise
S-44 Testing and using equipment
S-46 Anticipating and evaluating the effects of pharmacological and anesthetic agents
S-47 Documenting maintenance of a safe environment
S-48 Detecting significant changes in the environment
S-49 Preparing and handling specimens for diagnostic evaluation
S-50 Adapting to special and unusual needs
S-51 Identifying and communicating changes in patient status
S-52 Documenting nursing interventions and patient response
S-53 Educating, mentoring, and supervising health care team members
S-54 Recognizing impaired behavior in patients, family, and staff and responding appropriately
S-55 Recognizing personal limitations and seeking assistance as needed
S-56 Measuring, evaluating, and documenting patient outcomes
S-62 Setting priorities
S-64 Incorporating feedback into nurse performance
S-65 Applying ethical principles
S-67 Evaluating for signs and symptoms of injury
S-68 Performing required counts
S-69 Recording devices implanted or explanted during procedures
S-71 Securing patient belongings and valuables

PERIOPERATIVE NURSING INTERVENTIONS AND ACTIVITIES

Assessment to prevent physical injury is an ongoing activity that results in developing the nursing diagnosis and plan of care. Changes in the plan of care and interventions occur as necessary based on ongoing assessment criteria.

The perioperative nurse assesses both the patient and the environment. The initial patient assessment requires that the perioperative nurse understands the medical/surgical plan of care as it relates to the scheduled operative or invasive procedure, use and handling of equipment and supplies required for the procedure and the patient's physiological and psychological status. The environmental assessment requires that the perioperative nurse obtains, prepares, and verifies function of equipment and supplies that might be required. In addition, the perioperative nurse should examine the environment for equipment or conditions that pose a safety risk and take corrective action. Equipment and supplies that are infrequently used require competency validation to operate or use correctly.

The patient's individual uniqueness and the variability in procedures make it necessary to collect the data and impart knowledge and experiences to individualize the care. These critical thinking skills, problem solving, and decision making result in the patient focused and goal oriented outcomes.

The patient's medical record is a source of valuable information that can be used to identify needs based on the patient's condition. The patient's medical history and physical and laboratory reports provide baseline data for the assessment, nursing diagnosis, and care planning. The perioperative nurse should always review the patient's medical record for information including, but not limited to,

- patient identification;
- operative or invasive procedure, site, and side planned;

- history and physical including allergies (eg, medication, latex sensitivity), medication history, previous procedures, laboratory reports, and preexisting medical conditions.

The information gathered from the patient's record helps identify priority needs. The perioperative nurse can complete a patient assessment to verify accuracy and completeness of information and to determine specific or new details and risk factors (eg, skin integrity, extent of limitations, history of malignant hyperthermia, type of medication reactions) that can be used to determine nursing diagnosis.

The perioperative nurse communicates and documents patient assessment information, equipment or supplies that are required, nursing interventions, and adverse responses. The information is communicated to appropriate people depending on what information needs to be shared. Each person's knowledge related to the procedure and patient care needs influences correct decision making and interventions to provide comprehensive, patient-specific care. The perioperative nurse should communicate pertinent information to those providing care after surgery to increase their awareness of patient conditions and adverse responses that can occur after the patient is discharged from the operating room. Documentation provides a record of the patient's responses to care and baseline information for ongoing evaluation.

PREVENTING PHYSICAL INJURY

Extraneous Objects

Extraneous objects used during operative or other invasive procedures can include pneumatic tourniquets, compression devices, thermal regulation devices, and powered surgical instruments. Other objects include safety devices (eg, restraints, support devices), sponges, needles, sharps, instruments, and items that are small enough or have parts small enough to remain in a surgical incision after closure.

Items that could be retained in the patient should be accounted for before, during, and after the procedure. Items that come in parts or are broken during the procedure should be accounted for in totality. Items that are broken during a procedure are possibly required to be reported according to the institution's policies.

The perioperative nurse should be knowledgeable about the equipment, item, or device used for the procedure, including correct size and type needed for the procedure or patient and the correct use and handling according to the manufacturer's instructions. The perioperative nurse also should be aware of biomedical equipment inspections required for equipment and verify that it is completed as scheduled or when equipment is brought into the setting for single use. Supplies and equipment are selected based on the patient's needs and the planned operative or invasive procedure.

At minimum, patient assessment includes attention to the preoperative status of the integumentary, neuromuscular, and cardiovascular systems to prevent injury, impaired skin integrity, disturbed sensory perception, neurovascular dysfunction, or impaired physical mobility. Communication of status may be necessary because of the patient's condition or other information that is obtained that might alter the patient's response to treatment (eg, medications that were taken prior to surgery, such as aspirin or herbal therapies). The surgeon or anesthesia care provider may need to be notified or the plan of care modified, including the type of equipment or supplies planned to specifically meet the patient's needs.

Interventions that prevent injury from extraneous objects include, but are not limited to,

- identifies the patient, side, and site;
- implements protective measures to prevent skin or tissue injury due to thermal sources;
- implements protective measures to prevents skin/tissue injury due to mechanical sources;
- performs required counts;
- uses supplies and equipment within safe parameters;
- performs venipuncture; and
- maintains continuous surveillance of the patient and environment.

Institutional policies should be written and include guidelines for practice to protect the patient. For example, policies for cleaning and preparing equipment and supplies should identify practices used to verify function and integrity before repeat use for patient care. Employee competency should be validated for equipment and supplies that are infrequently used. Documentation of extraneous objects depends on the item, but most items used for therapeutic or treatment purposes are documented as used on the patient's record. This might include name of the item used, settings (eg, temperature, pressure), identification number, and length of time used. Documentation of counts includes the type of items accounted for, names and titles of personnel performing the counts, count results, and unusual circumstances that require the item to remain with the patient (eg, retained sponges for packing).

The patient is evaluated for signs and symptoms of physical injury to skin and tissue or other systems. The patient's skin is assessed for injury caused by sharp objects and equipment use (eg, tourniquet, electrocautery dispersive pad). The circulation, sensation, and motion of extremities is evaluated by inspecting color, size and shape, palpating for warmth, dryness and capillary refill, quality and volume of pulses, and complaints of pain or discomfort in areas other than that of the incision. Variances from expected findings are reported and documented.

Chemical Injury

Chemical injury can result because of incorrect use of chemicals, such as overexposure or inappropriate exposure. Chemicals include cleaning solutions, skin preparation solutions, methylmethacrylate, latex, or tissue preservatives. The perioperative nurse should be familiar with the information included on the Material Safety Data Sheet, product information on the container, and correct protocols for the use of chemicals.

At minimum, the patient assessment includes review of the integumentary, respiratory, cardiovascular, and gastrointestinal systems to prevent impaired skin integrity, ineffective breathing pattern, allergic response, nausea, or decreased cardiac output. The patient should be assessed for allergies or other adverse responses to agents such as adhesives, latex, iodine, and contrast media. The perioperative nurse must be familiar with chemical compounds and manufacturer's instructions for use. Because injury also can result when patients are sensitive to products such as latex, it is important to identify previous exposures. Patient assessment should include hypersensitivities or reactions to chemicals that could result in exposure to similar products or repeat exposure to the one being used. Family history can be indicative of the need to use chemicals with caution, particularly when caring for a child.

Personnel should be familiar with routines for mixing, cleaning, rinsing, drying, or fume evacuation to prevent unnecessary exposure of the patient to chemical agents that can be used to clean, disinfect, or prepare equipment or supplies (eg, OR bed, instruments), sterilize instruments, or clean the patient's incision site. Chemicals always should be used according to the manufacturer's instructions and should not be combined unless safe outcomes can be ensured.

Guidelines should be in place that will prevent patient exposure to residual chemicals after cleaning, disinfecting, or sterilizing equipment and supplies. This includes guidelines for a latex safe environment. Personnel should know the emergency procedures to be initiated in the event of a spill or unexpected exposure. Other nursing interventions include, but are not limited to,

- implements protective measures to prevent skin and tissue injury due to chemical sources;
- verifies allergies;
- implements latex allergy precautions as needed; and
- applies chemical hemostatic agents.

Patients are evaluated for allergic type responses to prep solutions, and skin integrity is inspected for redness, rash, abrasion, or blistering that can result from chemical exposure. Dependent areas of the body that might be exposed to prep solution because of pooling are inspected. In addition, the patient's respiratory status should be evaluated for signs and symptoms such as dyspnea, shortness of breath, labored respirations, wheezing, or stridor.

Electrical Injury

Electrical injury can result from faulty equipment or incorrect use or handling of the equipment. Patient conditions such as nutritional malnourishment with small muscle mass, those who have had implanted medical devices or other conditions also can be a precursor to electrical injury. At minimum, the patient's integumentary, neuromuscular, and cardiovascular status as well as pain perception should be assessed to prevent impaired skin integrity or acute pain. Assessing the patient's condition will alert the perioperative nurse to any possible changes in the plan of care. For example, if the patient has bony prominences, scar tissue, metal implants, or hairy skin surfaces, it is important to evaluate appropriate placement of the electrosurgical dispersive pad.

The priority nursing intervention includes, but is

not limited to, implementing protective measures to prevent injury due to electrical sources (eg, electrosurgery safety precautions, dispersive patient electrode safety precautions, active electrode safety precautions). Electrical equipment should be used according to the manufacturer's instructions and inspected prior to each use. Audible or visual alarm systems on equipment should be checked routinely to detect equipment fault. Biomedical equipment inspection also must be completed on a scheduled basis and equipment maintained. The perioperative nurse must be familiar with the principles of electrical safety as it relates to use of an electrosurgical unit, pacemaker, nerve stimulator, defibrillators, or electrical powered equipment.

The patient is evaluated for redness, blistering, or burns to the skin at the site of the patient dispersive electrode, bony prominences, or pressure sites. Changes in skin and tissue integrity are documented and reported to the health care providers who will be continuing care delivery.

Transfer/Transport

Transfer occurs when a patient is moved from one place to another (eg, to or from a bed to stretcher, the stretcher to OR bed) with assistance or aids. Transport occurs when a patient is moved via a device, such as wheelchair, stretcher or wagon (eg, for a child), bed, or when a patient ambulates with or without assistance. Within reasonable limits, patients should be allowed as much independence as possible during the processes. The transporter should ensure transfer without tissue injury, altered body temperature, ineffective breathing patterns, altered tissue perfusion, and undue discomfort, pain, or fear.

Transfer and/or transport injuries can occur when transport devices are not used correctly, the correct number of people are not available to assist, people are not familiar with transport procedures, or the transfer results in a fall, fracture, neuromuscular injury, or hypovolemia. In addition, patient transfer can result in skin damage from shearing or abrading injury if the patient is not moved correctly and with caution. If not protected and managed during transfer and transport, damage to peripheral sites such as those for infusion, urinary catheters, nasogastric tubes, chest tubes, or other devices also can occur. Tubes should be secured and tight, not kinked or placed beneath the patient, or allowed to totally infuse before another source can be added. Transport and transfer of patients on a ventilator or receiving oxygen, in traction, or who are medically unstable or unconscious should be completed by people knowledgeable in managing the equipment as well as able to manage critical patient care situations should they occur. Children should be transported via transport equipment or carried by the parent. If equipment is needed for the transport, it is important to ensure that battery power is adequate (eg, cardiac monitor) or leads and monitoring devices are secured (eg, pulse oxymeter).

At minimum, the perioperative nurse should assess the patient's integumentary system, musculoskeletal, cardiovascular, respiratory, and mental status as well as pain perception to prevent impaired skin integrity or risk for falls. Physical limitations including congenital deformities, changes caused by disease processes (eg, metastasis, edema, trauma), pain, and implanted devices should be identified.

The perioperative nurse should assess the patient's needs before transport to determine the necessary skill level and assign the personnel to transport. The correct transport devices must be obtained considering the patient's size and critical needs related to their condition, such as a casted extremity or oxygen administration. Specific transfer devices also are made available considering the individual patient's needs. Patients who are obese might require transport devices that will accommodate large patients or additional assistance may be required and should be planned. In addition, the transporter should be familiar with the equipment used for transport and transfer as well as critical situations that can arise during the processes so that they can be prepared to provide assistance or care as needed.

The appropriate number of people should be available to transfer and transport a patient. Patients transferred to or from the OR bed and are unable to assist with the transfer should be assisted by a minimum of four people including one person on each side, one person at the head, and one person at the foot. The transfer requires that one person directs the transfer and activities of others. Patient movement devices may be useful. Transfer and transport should be accomplished in a controlled fashion to prevent adverse outcomes such as shearing injury, change in cardiac status or pain. Efforts should be made to maintain the patient's temperature and protect privacy. Body alignment should be maintained, and the patient should be informed of actions related to the transfer or transport. Transport devices should be equipped with locking wheels and side rails. Side rails are elevated and secured in an upright position when moving a patient. It is suggested that one safety restraint should be placed across the upper body and one on the lower body of patients when being transferred. Transfer and transport devices should be stabilized and placed in the locked position when in use or at any time that they are not in use.

Following each transfer or transport, the patient should be evaluated for

- signs and symptoms of injury to the skin and tissue including redness, bruising, abrasion, compression, and/or pressure related to transport;
- vital signs within normal limits including temperature;
- changes in pain perception using the approved pain scale; or
- other possible adverse outcomes associated with transfer and transport (eg, patent infusion and drainage lines, dressings intact).

Positioning Injury

Proper positioning can decrease postoperative discomfort, expedite the operative or invasive procedure, and eliminate postoperative complications. Positioning injuries include tissue or skin damage, nerve injury, musculoskeletal changes, or compromise of other body systems. Positioning is a shared responsibility of the anesthesia care provider, surgeon, and perioperative nurse who might delegate the actions to others assisting with care of the patient. The care provided by each is a result of needs dependent on the other. The perioperative nurse identifies physical alterations that require additional precautions for procedure-specific positioning. Positions most commonly used for surgical procedures include

- supine,
- lithotomy,
- lateral,
- Trendelenburg,
- reverse Trendelenburg,
- prone, and
- sitting or semi-sitting.

Preventing injury requires that the perioperative nurse

- complete a thorough patient assessment to identify those at risk;
- transfer, transport, and position using body mechanics for self and to maintain the patient's alignment;
- recognize potential adverse effects related to the surgical procedure and anesthesia; and
- correctly use positioning equipment and supplies.

At minimum, the perioperative nurse should assess the patient's skin condition, cardiovascular, and neuromuscular status to identify risks for injury considering the planned procedure. Risks can include impaired skin integrity, perioperative positioning injury, impaired physical mobility, ineffective protection, and inadequate tissue perfusion. Prosthetics or corrective devices (eg, implants, pacemakers, hearing augmentation devices), presence of external devices (eg, drains, immobilizers), and patient specific conditions (eg, amputated body part, bone metastasis, trauma, congenital deformities) should be assessed to identify potential needs related to positioning.

The assessment should include visual observation of mobility and range of motion as it relates to the written physical or information reported by the patient. The patient's nutritional status and deficiencies also should be considered when assessing the positioning needs. The quality of peripheral pulses should be assessed when a patient is to be positioned in a manner that could interfere with circulation to the extremity. The perioperative nurse must understand the physiological responses as a result of the anesthetic agents or the surgical procedure.

The interventions provided by the perioperative nurse include, but are not limited to,

- identifies physical alterations that require additional precautions for procedure-specific positioning;
- verifies presence of prosthetics or corrective devices; and
- positions the patient to prevent neuromuscular injury, maintain skin and tissue integrity, and maintain body alignment and optimal physiological functioning.

It is the perioperative nurse's responsibility to meet patient needs through constant surveillance regarding safety concerns; continually assess and protect the patient throughout the procedure; modify the position as needed; and evaluate the position in the event it is changed during the procedure to prevent complications. The position selected for the patient should

- promote optimum exposure to the operative site while sustaining perfusion and respiratory function,
- maintain body alignment,
- prevent nerve damage, and
- preserve the patient's dignity.

The correct type and size of positioning devices must be obtained based on the patient's identified needs and planned operative or invasive procedure. The device function and cleanliness should be verified before use. Devices that require repair or replacement should be removed from service and not used for patient care. Positioning devices can include, but are not limited to,

- armboards,
- anesthesia screen,
- stirrups,
- headrest,
- footboard or extension,
- safety belt or restraints,
- lift sheet,
- shoulder or axillary roll, and
- padding for extremities or vulnerable sites, such as bony prominences or areas of circulatory compromise.

In addition, the procedure might require use of additional aids, such as antiembolitic stockings, elastic bandages, or pneumatic compression devices if the patient's legs will be in a dependent position for a long period of time or if the procedure increases the risk for compromise of a system.

Before anesthesia administration, the patient's comfort and functional limitations can be verified in supine or modified supine positions by asking the patient to assume the position that will be used during the surgery. If the patient is awake, he or she is informed and should assume the position planned for the procedure. The patient's response to the position is evaluated and the position adapted to accommodate limitations. General considerations regarding intraoperative transfer and positioning include, but are not limited to, the following.

- Body parts should be moved within their normal range of motion in a slow, gradual manner.
- Body alignment, including alignment of the legs (ie, uncrossed position), must be maintained.
- Extremities (eg, fingers), nerves, and external devices must be protected.
- Mobility limitations of the patient and natural body alignment determine the extent of position possible for the procedure.
- Attachments should be placed on the opposite side of the operative bed prior to transfer from a stretcher to prevent interference with the transfer.
- Anesthesia should be administered prior to positioning.
- Awake patients should be informed prior to and assist with positioning activities when possible.

After the patient is positioned, they should be secured so that there is not an unplanned change in the position during the procedure. Safety belts or other devices are placed securely, but not so tight that blood flow or nerve function is compromised. The patient is monitored throughout the procedure for external pressures (eg, instruments, leaning) that might be applied by members of the health care team. If repositioning occurs, the patient and positioning devices are again checked for placement and security. The perioperative nurse documents position and positioning changes as well as the patient's condition as it relates to risk for positioning injury.

The perioperative nurse evaluates for signs and symptoms of injury that can result from positioning by examining the patient to assess peripheral pulses and neuromuscular impairments; sites related to positioning devices for skin and tissue integrity; pressure areas for signs of skin injury; and vital signs within normal limits. At minimum, the adverse outcomes are documented in addition to the patient's position and interventions to meet specific patient care needs.

Laser Injury

Laser safety is a responsibility of all team members throughout an operative or invasive procedure. It is intended that the patient receives the minimal laser energy exposure needed to achieve the therapeutic purpose and has no contact with the laser beam other than for the intended purpose. Tissue interaction that can occur when using medical lasers includes electromechanical, photoablative, thermal, and photochemical. The most common laser found in operating rooms is the carbon dioxide laser. Others include the yttrium aluminum garnet (YAG), potassium titanyl phosphate (KTP), argon, excimer, and tunable dye lasers.

At minimum, patients will be assessed for integumentary integrity, visual and pain perception, and neuromuscular and musculoskeletal status for risk of impaired skin integrity, pain, disturbed sensory perception, or altered functional status. Laser injury can occur as an emergent situation if safety precautions have not been implemented and monitored. The perioperative nurse must be educated about the type of laser being used and the procedure being performed. Caution should be taken to implement safety precautions appropriate for the type of laser used.

A laser safety officer should be assigned to monitor correct use and handling of lasers between and during procedures and to manage protocols for education and use by employees and surgeons. Each laser type requires education and training so that the user and the operator can safely deliver the laser treatment. Protective measures for employees and patients are mandated during laser use.

The type of protective measures varies with the type of laser and procedure planned. Laser precautions can include

- teaching the patient protective techniques, such as not wearing make-up and hair spray;
- protecting the eyes using appropriate methods (eg, using a water-based lubricant, taping the eyelids closed, covering with secured moist eye pads and a very moist sterile towel, placing soft goggles appropriate for the laser wavelength after taping the eyelids, using corneal shields);
- protecting the area around the surgical site by placing water or saline saturated towels or sponges;
- using the correct endotracheal tube for the laser procedure;
- using caution when oxygen is administered during laser use;
- eliminating use of flammable solutions;
- using anodized, ebonized, dull surfaced, nonreflective, or matte-finished instruments;
- placing backstops or guards to prevent the laser beam from striking the normal tissue;
- using a laser plume evacuation system;
- understanding emergency procedures, location of emergency equipment, and laser safety precautions; and
- maintaining the laser in standby mode or "off" position when not in use.

Personnel should be familiar with the type of laser being used and precautions for use so that they can protect themselves and the patient. Limiting access to the surgical suite, covering windows, providing and wearing safety eyewear, and placing laser safety signs at the entrances of laser treatment areas are some precautions that should be taken.

Patients are evaluated for laser injury by observing for injury unrelated to the intended therapeutic effects of the laser therapy. The skin and adjacent tissue is inspected and assessed for discolored, reddened, raised, or painful areas. Patients also are assessed for vision difficulty and instructed to report complaints of visual problems or headaches after surgery.

Radiation Injury

Patients should be free from signs and symptoms of radiation injury after an operative or other invasive procedure. They should be exposed to radiation only if it is medically indicated. Radiation injury can result when patients are not properly protected from unnecessary radiation exposure. Radiation is classified into three categories, of which two can pose a threat to personnel and patients. Primary radiation (ie, that resulting from a beam) and secondary radiation (ie, that resulting when the primary beam interacts with the patient or an object and is deflected or partially absorbed) can potentially result in injury. The third type, remnant radiation, poses little threat to personnel; it is the radiation that exits the patient to produce an image on film.

Patients may be exposed to radionuclides for diagnostic or therapeutic purposes. Radionuclide materials are absorbed by the body, but until that occurs the patients may emit radiation. Personnel who are transporting patients who received radionucides should be aware of precautions, and advance communication with areas where the patient will be transported is necessary.

Radium implants should be handled with precautionary measures by a person who is knowledgeable about the safety factors. Body fluids or tissue removed from a patient who has undergone radiation therapy should be transferred in a safe manner. Guidelines for contamination control measures should be implemented.

Distance, shielding, and time are the most common methods of protection from radiation. Because patients cannot maintain a distance, it is important that shielding be used correctly to protect from unnecessary radiation exposure. The standard thickness for shielding for radiation protection is 0.25 inches. Leaded shields should be used to protect the patient's ovaries or testes, thyroid, and the fetus if a pregnant woman requires radiation exposure.

Radiation exposure can occur from fluoroscopy (c-arm) equipment, radiographic (x-ray) equipment, or radium implants. Exposure is limited if personnel understand the use of protective equipment, vulnerable tissue or areas of the body, and correct use of the equipment. Personnel who operate radiation equipment must be trained specifically for that equipment use.

Nursing interventions include, but are not limited to,

- assesses patients at minimum for previous radiological exposure, cognition, and predisposing skin conditions to prevent impaired skin integrity, confusion, or unnecessary exposure; and
- implements protective measures to prevent injury due to radiation sources.

Premenopausal women should have a pregnancy test before procedures with radiation. Protective equipment including leaded patient shields for the gonads and thyroid should be placed anytime that radiation will be used, even for a short period of time. The perioperative nurse documents the measures used to protect the patient.

Following the operative or invasive procedure, the patient's skin and tissue should be observed for signs of changes including redness, abrasions, bruising, blistering, or edema. Variances from the expected appearance are reported and documented.

Medication Administration

Medication administration occurs via oral, intravenous, topical, or intramuscular routes in the perioperative setting. Guidelines for therapies such as transfusion administration and emergency treatments such as malignant hyperthermia should be implemented as well as other medication administration guidelines.

The perioperative nurse must be knowledgeable about medications that patients routinely take, as well as those ordered for the operative or invasive procedure. The patient's culturally based home health remedies and herbal therapies also should be revealed and the influence on medication management determined. It is the responsibility of the perioperative nurse to administer the correct medication and dosage to the correct patient at the correct time via the correct route. A medication that is correctly delivered at the incorrect time (eg, preoperative antibiotic therapy, anticlotting agents) might not result in an obvious injury, but can result in an adverse outcome when the patient does not receive the medication correctly. The perioperative nurse should be familiar with current and reliable medication references.

The patient's integumentary and cognitive status should be assessed to prevent risk of injury. The patient also should be able to state that they understand the purpose, effects, and side effects of medications administered.

Interventions implemented by the perioperative nurse to prevent medication injury include, but are not limited to,

- verifies allergies including idiosyncrasises and sensitivities to medications, foods, and chemical agents;
- prescribes medications within the scope of practice; and

- administers prescribed medications and solutions.

Additional safety interventions by perioperative nurses to prevent medication injury include verifying medication labels and medications delivered to the sterile field with another professional practitioner including medication, strength, dosage, and expiration date; labeling medications on and off of the field; and communicating medication strength and dosage as the medication is passed to the person who will administer the medication.

The patient is evaluated for response to medications. The perioperative nurse observes for response and adverse reactions to medications administered and monitors patients for signs of the therapeutic effect, allergic effects, or toxicity. The patient's understanding of the potential complications or interactions also is evaluated. Signs and symptoms of adverse reactions are reported to the appropriate member of the health care team.

SUMMARY

Preventing physical injury is a responsibility of multiple health care providers because of the extent and degree of caution that must be considered when using equipment and supplies to provide patient care. Although the RN is not responsible for delivering all interventions, he or she must be aware of what should and should not be delegated to other team members to achieve safe outcomes. The perioperative nurse has unlimited responsibilities to create a culture of safety as they coordinate and manage the activities of people providing the care to accomplish the expected outcomes and prevent adverse events. Their priorities are to access the information, know and understand patient's needs, and focus on those interventions that require critical thinking to provide individualized care. Competencies in assessment, diagnosing, planning, intervening, and evaluating are basic skills that must be developed if the RN is to improve outcomes. In addition, perioperative nurses' experiences and skills are useful as the operative and invasive procedures continue to develop.

CASE STUDIES

Case Study: Mrs. H

Mrs. H is a 73-year-old white female admitted to the OR for repair of a fractured hip. She appears quite frail (5'5", 112 lbs), and you note that she has abrasions on her face and arms, in addition to her fractured right hip, which were sustained in a fall down the stairs at home. The admitting notes state that she is diabetic. Currently she controls her diabetes with diet and oral medication. She also has been diagnosed with osteoporosis and has had a previous wrist fracture from a fall. She lives alone but is accompanied by her daughter who lives near her. She appears to be in pain but is alert and oriented.

Points to Consider

- How does Mrs. H's injury and concurrent diagnoses affect her potential for physical injury during the perioperative period?
- How does Mrs. H's diabetes and osteoporosis affect her potential for healing?
- What nursing interventions will you use to prevent further patient injury?
- How can you alter your nursing care to protect this patient during her surgical experience?

Discussion of Points to Consider

Mrs. H is at risk for potential injury due to transfer, transport, and positioning because of her injuries, frail condition, and osteoporosis. Diabetes affects tissue perfusion, sensation, and healing. Osteoporosis affects the body's ability to repair bone and can render the patient at increased risk for further bone fractures or bone degeneration. Mrs. H is at risk for electrical and chemical injury because of her current skin condition, injuries, and diabetes. Extraneous objects in use during her procedure (eg, thermal regulating devices, the fracture table, powered surgical instruments) can also contribute to injury in an elderly, frail patient.

The nurse alters his or her plan of care to include the following:

- Careful questioning of the patient and gentle assessment is needed to determine how much range of motion is possible, where the patient is injured, and what areas require altered positioning, padding, or protection.
- Careful assessment of skin and documentation of injuries.
- Gathering of needed padding and safety devices.
- Alerting of personnel needed for transfer or positioning.
- Assessment of allergies or skin sensitivities to prevent the potential for chemical injury.
- Smoothing of all sheets/material under the patient, padding of pressure points, protection of injured areas, correct body alignment within

patient's ability to move.

- Discussion and documentation of all positioning difficulties with surgeon and anesthesia care personnel.
- Careful assessment of the patient following the surgical procedure and documentation of her condition upon leaving the OR to ensure no injury has occurred.

Case Study: Mr. JW

JW is a 32-year-old black male who stands 5'4" tall and weighs 215 lbs. He is admitted to the preoperative area for a gastric stapling procedure. He has been on a weight loss program for one year and has lost 100 lbs. Because of his weight, he has led a very sedentary life. He has arthritis in both knees and hips and is hypertensive. You note that his overall skin condition is poor and the admitting nurse has noted a "reddened area" on his sacrum while helping him to undress. He is able to walk, but with much exertion. His blood pressure is 160/90 despite medication. He appears anxious and is accompanied by his mother who is also quite overweight and anxious.

Points to Consider

- What potential injuries is this patient at risk for and why?
- How can you prevent these potential injuries?
- What assessments and interventions can you make perioperatively, and how do you document their success or failure?

Discussion of Points to Consider

The perioperative nurse is aware that this patient is at risk for injury during transport, transfer, and positioning. There is risk for injury from chemicals and extraneous objects in the OR and electrical injury. JW's obesity, arthritis and its resulting decreased range of motion, and hypertension make skin care, positioning, and protection and padding of extremities and pressure points essential. Due to his obesity and subsequent weight loss, his overall nutritional status may be altered; thus, he is at risk for skin breakdown and delayed healing.

In his or her plan of care, the nurse:

- Assesses the patient for potential areas of risk. In this case, he or she assesses the "reddened area over his sacrum," the patient's overall skin condition and range of motion, noting his limitations and re-evaluating how these will affect positioning and the need for protective padding.
- Assembles OR bed extensions or positioning devices and protective padding and restraints. He or she requests transfer help and plans the transfer of the patient to the OR bed in consultation with the surgeon, the anesthesia care provider, and other perioperative personnel who will be assisting. Positioning the patient awake on the OR bed if possible helps to ensure his comfort and prevent injury. The nurse obtains antiembolic stockings or pneumatic compression devices for use.
- Ensures that all sheets are smoothed and any excess prep solutions are removed and not allowed to pool on or under the patient or in skin folds.

In the immediate postoperative period, the nurse can assess the patient's skin condition paying special attention to pressure points, skin folds, and the skin under the electrosurgical unit grounding pad. He or she documents the findings. The patient should not experience any pain or discomfort as a result of positioning, transfer, or the use of extraneous objects in the OR; his pain should be confined to the surgical site.

SUGGESTED LEARNING ACTIVITIES

- ◆ Review AORN's *Standards, Recommended Practices, and Guidelines* and the *Perioperative Nursing Data Set.*

- ◆ Review your institution's policies and procedures regarding nursing care plans and the documentation of nursing diagnoses, interventions, and outcomes.

- ◆ Practice making nursing care plans and reviewing your current nursing care plans to evaluate your strengths and weaknesses in preventing injury. In what areas do you need the most practice?

- ◆ Review perioperative nursing texts (eg, *Alexander's Care of the Patient in Surgery, Berry & Kohn's Operating Room Technique, Care of the Patient During Operative and Invasive Procedures*) for further information regarding preventing injury during the perioperative experience.

- ◆ Review the patient care provided in cases where an injury has occurred. How could the injury have been anticipated or prevented? What would you do differently? What care was appropriate or inappropriate?

- Practice identifying patients at increased risk for injury and draw up nursing care plans that address those issues.

- What, in general, do you need to improve your routine care of patients to prevent injury?

RECOMMENDED STUDY MATERIALS

AORN, "Competency Statements in Perioperative Nursing," in *Standards, Recommended Practices, and Guidelines* (Denver: AORN, Inc, 2002) 19-21.

AORN, "AORN Guidance Statement—Safe Medication Practices in Perioperative Settings," *AORN Journal* 75 (May 2002) 1008-1009; http://www.patient safetyfirst.org/guidancestatement.pdf.

AORN, "AORN Position Statement on Correct Site Surgery," in *Standards, Recommended Practices, and Guidelines* (Denver: AORN, Inc, 2002) 123-125.

AORN, "Recommended Practices for Documentation of Perioperative Nursing Care," in *Standards, Recommended Practices, and Guidelines* (Denver: AORN, Inc, 2002) 217-219.

AORN, "Recommended Practices for Electrosurgery," in *Standards, Recommended Practices, and Guidelines* (Denver: AORN, Inc, 2002) 221-228.

AORN, "Recommended Practices for High-Level Disinfection," in *Standards, Recommended Practices, and Guidelines* (Denver: AORN, Inc, 2002) 211-216.

AORN, "Recommended Practices for Laser Safety in Practice Settings," in *Standards, Recommended Practices, and Guidelines* (Denver: AORN, Inc, 2002) 277-281.

AORN, "Recommended Practices for Safe Care Through Identification of Potential Hazards in the Surgical Environment," in *Standards, Recommended Practices, and Guidelines* (Denver: AORN, Inc, 2002) 261-266.

AORN, "Recommended Practices for Sponge, Sharp, and Instrument Counts," in *Standards, Recommended Practices, and Guidelines* (Denver: AORN, Inc, 2002) 205-210.

AORN, "Recommended Practices for Use of the Pneumatic Tourniquet," in *Standards, Recommended Practices, and Guidelines* (Denver: AORN, Inc, 2002) 293-298.

AORN, "Standards of Perioperative Nursing," in *Standards, Recommended Practices, and Guidelines* (Denver: AORN, Inc, 2002) 153154.

Beyea, S, ed, *Perioperative Nursing Data Set*, second ed (Denver: AORN, Inc, 2002).

Davis, B, "Perioperative care of patients with latex allergy," *AORN Journal* 72:1 (2000) 47-54.

Meeker, M H; Rothrock, J D, eds, *Alexander's Care of the Patient in Surgery*, 12th ed (St Louis: Mosby, Inc, 2002).

Shymko, M; Shymko T M, "Radiation safety," *AORN Journal* 68 (October 1998) 596-602.

CHAPTER 6: IMPLEMENT PLAN OF CARE TO OPTIMIZE PHYSIOLOGICAL PROTECTION

Robin Chard, RN, MSN, CNOR

Patient assessment is the first step of the nursing process and involves gathering data through the health history and physical examination. Data is collected in a systematic manner using a problem-solving approach to identify actual or potential health problems. A relationship between the patient and nurse is started to elicit quality information and develop a relationship of mutual respect and trust. Active patient involvement in the assessment phase is necessary to secure effective therapeutic communication.

Assessment data may be derived from several sources. Aside from the health history and assessment, the nurse obtains information by interviewing the patient's family or significant others and reviewing the medical chart. The nurse is able to organize, examine, analyze, and synthesize the collected data into a workable whole, which is then communicated to members of the health care team as needed.

The nursing diagnosis follows the initial assessment and includes identifying specific problems or complications that require collaborative interventions. A plan of care is established to develop goals, prioritize care, and establish expected outcomes. The implementation phase puts the plan of nursing care into action through collective efforts of the health care team members, including documentation of care.

This chapter emphasizes the implementation phase of the nursing process to optimize physiological protection of a patient during a surgical or invasive procedure.

LEARNING OBJECTIVES

1. Identify potential and real risks for physiological alterations.
2. List measures to minimize physiological alterations.
3. Determine nursing interventions to control for physiologic alterations in the cardiovascular, pulmonary, neurological, and integumentary systems, including body temperature maintenance and fluid and electrolyte balance.
4. Modify plan of care as needed to optimize physiological protection.

TASK STATEMENT; AREAS OF KNOWLEDGE AND SKILL

Task Statement

Optimize physiological protection by minimizing risk for infection and by maintaining/improving wound/tissue perfusion; body temperature; fluid and electrolyte balance; and pulmonary, cardiac, and neurological status.

Areas of Knowledge

K-1 Health assessment techniques
K-2 Anatomy and physiology
K-3 Pathophysiology
K-4 Pharmacology and anesthetic agents
K-5 Pain management
K-6 Principles of wound healing
K-7 Diagnostic procedures and results
K-8 Preoperative patient preparation activities
K-9 Surgical, anesthetic, and other perioperative interventions
K-11 Physiologic responses to the surgical experience
K-12 Principles of positioning
K-13 Ergonomics and body mechanics
K-14 Transfer and transport techniques and equipment

K-15 Risks for injury, including but not limited to, skin, positioning, and retained foreign body
K-16 Emergency procedures (eg, CPR, MH)
K-17 Postoperative complications
K-18 Defining characteristics of impending patient physiologic crisis
K-19 Emergency operative procedures
K-21 Communication theories and techniques
K-23 Discharge planning
K-25 *Perioperative Nursing Data Set* (PNDS)
K-27 Microbiology and infection control
K-28 Standard and transmission-based precautions
K-29 Potential hazards in the perioperative environment including, but not limited to, chemical, electrical, fire, gas, laser, physical environment, radiologic, and extraneous objects
K-30 Interventions to optimize safety
K-31 Technologies and equipment relating to perioperative practice
K-32 Environmental parameters (eg, temperature, humidity, air exchange)
K-33 Principles of sterilization and disinfection
K-34 Protective barrier materials
K-35 Packaging materials
K-36 Principles of equipment inspection, maintenance, and repair
K-42 Nursing research and evidence based practice
K-44 Regulatory standards and voluntary guidelines
K-45 AORN *Standards, Recommended Practices, and Guidelines*
K-46 AORN position statements (eg, bloodborne pathogens, do-not-resuscitate orders [DNR])
K-47 Principles of problem solving
K-50 Defining characteristics of impaired individuals (eg, substance abuse, psychological disturbance, compromised performance)
K-53 Rules, responsibilities, and duties of health care team members and internal and external support service personnel
K-56 Implants (eg, handling, tracking, sterilization)

Areas of Skill

S-1 Confirming patient identity, operative site, and procedure
S-2 Collecting, analyzing, and prioritizing patient data
S-3 Using health assessment techniques (eg, interview, observation, auscultation, palpation, percussion)
S-4 Communicating effectively (verbal and nonverbal)
S-5 Advocating and protecting patient rights
S-6 Evaluating environment for discharge care
S-7 Assessing and managing pain
S-8 Assessing for potential abuse (eg, substance, domestic)
S-9 Assessing readiness to learn, knowledge level, and preferred learning style
S-11 Identifying risk of infection and injury
S-12 Identifying cultural, spiritual, and ethnic issues of care
S-13 Identifying age specific needs
S-14 Formulating a nursing diagnosis
S-15 Collaborating with other members on the health care team
S-16 Applying AORN *Standards, Recommended Practices, and Guidelines*
S-17 Applying the *Perioperative Nursing Data Set* (PNDS)
S-18 Delineating and communicating measurable patient outcomes
S-19 Participating in quality improvement activities
S-20 Maintaining accurate patient records
S-22 Providing evidence based care
S-23 Applying regulatory standards and voluntary guidelines
S-24 Developing a patient and family education plan
S-26 Incorporating community and institutional resources into plan of care
S-28 Adapting to changing situations and technologies
S-29 Performing nursing interventions
S-30 Documenting all relevant facts and data elements with appropriate terminology
S-31 Recording unusual occurrences and/or variances in care
S-33 Anticipating the needs for equipment, supplies, and personnel
S-35 Maintaining the dignity, modesty, and privacy of the patient and protecting the confidentiality of patient information
S-36 Applying principles of aseptic technique and infection control
S-37 Applying principles of sterilization and disinfection
S-38 Applying principles of environmental cleaning
S-39 Maintaining a sterile field
S-40 Preparing the surgical site
S-41 Selecting appropriate protective barrier materials
S-42 Conducting biological monitoring
S-43 Controlling environmental noise
S-44 Testing and using equipment
S-45 Monitoring physiological parameters
S-46 Anticipating and evaluating the effects of pharmacological and anesthetic agents
S-47 Documenting maintenance of a safe environment
S-48 Detecting significant changes in the environment
S-49 Preparing and handling specimens for diagnostic

evaluation
S-50 Adapting to special and unusual needs
S-51 Identifying and communicating changes in patient status
S-52 Documenting nursing interventions and patient response
S-54 Recognizing impaired behavior in patients, family, and staff members and responding appropriately
S-55 Recognizing personal limitations and seeking assistance as needed
S-57 Performing sterilization procedures and conducting monitoring techniques (eg, chemical, biological monitoring, mechanical indicators)
S-58 Identifying appropriate packaging materials for sterilization
S-59 Selecting appropriate and cost-effective sterilization methods
S-60 Directing health care team members in emergency situations
S-61 Performing basic life support and other emergency procedures
S-62 Setting priorities
S-65 Applying ethical principles
S-70 Classifying the surgical wound

PERIOPERATIVE NURSING ACTIVITIES

A perioperative assessment is essential if nursing interventions are to be successful and appropriate. Identifying pre-existing diseases and risk factors will help the nurse develop an individualized plan of care for each patient. Interventions based on sound clinical judgment and knowledge will help the nurse optimize and protect the patient's physiological state. The nurse should be aware of the following areas of physiological concern throughout the perioperative phase:

- ◆ minimizing the patient's risk of infection;
- ◆ maintaining or improving the patient's wound/tissue perfusion, body temperature, fluid and electrolyte balance, pulmonary status, cardiovascular status, and neurological status; and
- ◆ giving special attention to evaluating the risk status of gerontological, neonatal, and immunocompromised patients.

Preoperative Phase

During the preoperative phase, the nurse should assess the patient's risks in each of the following categories.

- ◆ Minimize Risk of Infection
  - Disease processes, laboratory values, medication use, hydration status, or other risk factors (eg, presence of immunosuppporesion that may increase risk for infection).
  - Baseline vital signs. Are there deviations that could compromise the patient's ability to fight infection?
  - Abnormal vs. normal laboratory values. Note abnormalities and assess their effects on risk for infection.
  - Preoperative assessment tool. Incorporate into your preoperative assessment.
  - Allergies or sensitivities. What are the patient's allergies or sensitivities, and do they compromise the immune system enough to increase the patient's risk for infection?
  - Preoperative skin preparation. What has been ordered, and how does that effect infection risk?
  - Antibiotic therapy. Has this been ordered? Has patient received prescribed medications?
  - Hygienic measures. What is the patient's general state of hygiene? Will it contribute to an increased risk of infection? How can you alter this?

- ◆ Maintain or Improve Wound/Tissue Perfusion
  - Does the patient have disease processes or factors that will increase the risk of altered tissue perfusion (eg, diabetes mellitus)?
  - If the patient is impaired in a way that will affect tissue perfusion, what is the patient's degree of impairment?
  - What is the patient's present physical status, and does it have any adverse effects on wound or tissue perfusion?
  - Nutritional status. Does the patient's nutritional status vary enough from normal to affect his or her ability to perfuse or heal tissue?
  - Noninvasive or invasive measures. What has been done, and what is planned? How will it affect tissue perfusion?
  - Laboratory values and diagnostic tools. Have these measures revealed any information that will affect tissue perfusion?
  - Baseline data. Establish baseline data and assess for risks.
  - Presence of dehydration, hypovolemia, electrolyte imbalances. Assess for these conditions and plan how they will affect the patient and how they can be corrected.

- Body temperature
  - Baseline data. Assess the patient and note deviations from baseline.
  - What factors may alter the patient's body temperature during this phase of care?
  - What is the patient's physical status?
  - What has your physical assessment told you about the patient's ability to maintain his or her body temperature? What will you need to assist the patient?
  - How will you alter the surgical environment to meet the needs of the patient?

- Fluid and Electrolyte Balance
  - What is the patient's hydration status?
  - What parenteral methods are needed for hydration?
  - What is the patient's NPO status?
  - What is the patient's physical status?
  - Are the patient's baseline vital signs significant of any fluid or electrolyte imbalance?
  - What does the patient's skin reveal during your assessment?
  - Does the patient use drugs or alcohol that can affect fluid or electrolyte balance?

- Pulmonary Status
  - Health history. What affects the patient's pulmonary status (eg, smoking, chronic lung disease)?
  - Assess respiratory status. Is there underlying respiratory disease (eg, asthma, chronic obstructive pulmonary disease [COPD]) or infection? Is there cough present or other physical abnormalities suggestive of respiratory disease? Is there a chest x-ray? Are there blood gases, clinical information (eg, oxygen saturation), or other laboratory values that will help you assess the patient's lung function?
  - Promote optimal lung expansion (eg, teach deep breathing and coughing exercises)

- Cardiovascular Status
  - What does the patient's health history, physical examination, and baseline vital signs reveal about his or her cardiovascular status?
  - Is there evidence of underlying cardiovascular disease (eg, hypertension, peripheral vascular disease, stroke, thromboembolism)?
  - What do laboratory, electrocardiogram (ECG), oxygen saturation, or other diagnostic test results reveal?
  - What medications is the patient taking?
  - What does your assessment reveal about the patient's heart rate, peripheral pulses, neck veins, presence of edema, or skin abnormalities?
  - What supplies or equipment will you need to gather to assist the patient during the intraoperative phase?

- Neurological Status
  - What does an assessment of the patient reveal?
  - What does baseline data (eg, mental status, level of consciousness, communication skills, motor skills, emotional behavior) reveal?
  - Is there a health history of stroke, hypertension, seizures, headaches, or other neurological disorders?
  - How has the patient reacted to previous anesthetics?
  - Has there been drug or alcohol use?

Intraoperative Phase

Continuing assessment of the patient is required during the intraoperative phase in the following areas.

- Minimize Risk of Infection
  - Surgical asepsis must be maintained by the use of environmental controls, traffic pattern control, continuous surveillance, conscientious techniques, the use of personal protective equipment, the maintenance of the patient's skin integrity and classification of the patient's wound.

- Maintain or Improve Wound/ Tissue Perfusion
  - The use of proper positioning to maintain good lung function and ensure no compromise of cardiovascular or neurological status.
  - Precautionary measures for compromised patients (eg, elderly, thin, obese).
  - Continuous monitoring of cardiopulmonary status.
  - Identification of abnormal laboratory values related to the patient's status.
  - Monitor equipment and devices in use.
  - Report changes in the patient's vital signs and oxygenation status.

- Body Temperature
  - Monitor core body temperature, urinary

output, ECG, blood pressure, and serum electrolytes.
- Use thermoregulation devices to cool or warm patient as needed.
- Limit patient exposure.
- Control external room temperature.
- Supply appropriately warmed or cooled irrigation or parenteral fluids as needed.
- Use dry linens and blankets.
- Use airway humidifier.
- Minimize or reverse physiologic process of hypothermia.

◆ Fluid and Electrolyte Balance
- Monitor fluid volume including irrigation, urinary output, and vital signs.
- Monitor laboratory values.
- Monitor skin integrity (eg, turgor, temperature, presence of edema).
- Watch for signs and symptoms of fluid volume excess or deficit.
- Use blood or blood products to correct any imbalance.
- Document blood loss, amount of IV fluids, and irrigation.

◆ Pulmonary Status
- Assist anesthesia care provider with difficult airway.
- Monitor the patient for complications (eg, inadequate ventilation, airway compromise, hypoxia).
- Correct anatomical positioning to prevent compromised gas exchange.
- Monitor peripheral perfusion and pulse oximeter values.

◆ Cardiovascular Status
- Use correct anatomical positioning to prevent compromised cardiovascular status.
- Monitor vital signs, pulse oximeter values, the rate and amount of blood and fluid loss, and intake and output.
- Assess peripheral perfusion and pulses and the color of tissues and blood.
- Monitor laboratory values and devices in use.

◆ Neurological Status
- Correct anatomical positioning to prevent undue pressure on nerves.
- Institute safety interventions related to risk of injury (eg, history of stroke, other neurological deficits).
- Monitor vital signs and note any changes in mental status.
- Assess pain levels and institute pain management techniques.
- Assess reflexes and the patient's motor and sensory function.

Postoperative Phase

These same areas of assessment must be followed during the patient's postoperative phase to ensure the optimal experience and reduction of risk for the patient.

◆ Minimize Risk of Infection
- Institute wound care management to include assessment, prevention of contamination, and enhancement of healing.
- Use standard precautions to protect patient and staff members from disease transmission.
- Use medication therapy (eg, antibiotics) if prescribed.
- Use isolation techniques if required.

◆ Maintain or Improve Wound/Tissue Perfusion
- Monitor the patient's vital signs.
- Assess and manage the surgical wound site.
- Encourage and assist with early ambulation, proper positioning, and pain management.
- Monitor intake and output.

◆ Body Temperature
- Monitor the patient's temperature, vital signs, and cardiac function.
- Assess for signs and symptoms of hypothermia or hyperthermia.
- Manage the temperature of the patient's environment.
- Use external devices for temperature control.
- Monitor at-risk patients (eg, elderly, neonates) carefully.

◆ Fluid and Electrolyte Balance
- Monitor intake and output, laboratory values, vital signs, and fluid volume.
- Assess the patient's skin, IV site, fluid volume or deficits, and wound for complications relating to fluid imbalance.
- Replace fluids that are lost.
- Assess for nausea or vomiting.
- Institute medication therapy if needed.

- Pulmonary Status
  - Help the patient maintain a patent airway.
  - Monitor for hypoventilation.
  - Assess breath sounds, vital signs, and pulse oximetry.
  - Remove excess secretions and help the patient properly position himself or herself.
  - Institute pain management techniques.
  - Encourage deep breathing, coughing, and early ambulation.

- Cardiovascular Status
  - Monitor the patient's skin color, temperature, vital signs, and pulse oximetry.
  - Assess for peripheral pulses, dysrhythmias, hypotension, shock, hemorrhage, hypertension.
  - Monitor the patency of IV lines, intake and output, and fluid replacement.
  - Replace fluids.
  - Institute leg exercises and frequent position changes.
  - Use sequential compression devices or anti-embolism stockings.

- Neurological Status
  - Assess the patient's mental status, level of consciousness, motor and sensory ability, presence of paresthesias, peripheral pulses, and sensations.
  - Institute medication therapy and pain management.
  - Provide a safe environment.
  - Assess the patient using the Aldrete score criteria.
  - Assess the patient against the baseline values noted preoperatively and intraoperatively.

RECOMMENDED PRACTICES

The following AORN recommended practices relating to physiological protection of the patient should be reviewed.

- "Recommended Practices for Surgical Attire"
- "Recommended Practices for Managing the Patient Receiving Conscious Sedation/Analgesia"
- "Recommended Practices for Environmental Cleaning in the Surgical Practice Setting"
- "Recommended Practices for Environmental Responsibility"
- "Recommended Practices for Surgical Hand Scrubs"
- "Recommended Practices for Safe Care Through Identification of Potential Hazards in the Surgical Environment"
- "Recommended Practices for Use of the Pneumatic Tourniquet"
- "Recommended Practices for Positioning the Patient in the Perioperative Practice Setting"
- "Recommended Practices for Skin Preparation of Patients"
- "Recommended Practices for Maintaining a Sterile Field"
- "Recommended Practices for Traffic Patterns in the Perioperative Practice Setting"

SUMMARY

A perioperative nurse must be competent in the delivery of care related to the physiologic monitoring of the patient and optimizing physiological protection and safety. A working knowledge of the nursing process combined with the ability to carry out specific nursing interventions will contribute to a favorable patient outcome. Beginning with an assessment, the nurse collects data, forms a plan of care, implements the plan, and evaluates the care. The nursing process is a circular construct whereby the perioperative nurse continuously re-evaluates and adjusts nursing care according to the patient's needs.

CASE STUDIES

Case Study: Mr. P

A 40-year-old patient is scheduled for an exploratory laparotomy for possible splenectomy after a motor vehicle accident. The patient has two IV lines (#18g) and an indwelling urinary catheter in place and is receiving oxygen therapy via a non-rebreather mask. The patient has been immobilized on a backboard and is wearing a cervical collar. The patient is awake, oriented, and complaining of severe abdominal pain. What priorities of care are needed to optimize the patient's physiological protection?

Points to Consider

- Initial assessment includes airway, breathing status,

oxygen saturation, blood gases, laboratory data.
- Assessment of pulses (eg, distal extremities), blood pressure, capillary refill, cardiac rate and rhythm, skin color, and temperature.
- Fluid replacement measures, intake and output, urine characteristics.
- Maintain correct body position to keep stabilization of cervical spine.
- Assess neurological status, including level of consciousness, behavior, and motor and sensory function.
- Perform pulse, movement, and sensation on extremities.
- Any pre-existing disease/illness.
- Laboratory/diagnostic tests to consider include: urinalysis, complete blood count, chemistry, arterial blood gases, type and screen for blood, x-rays, ECG, CT scan.

Nursing Diagnoses

- Ineffective breathing pattern
- Fluid volume deficit
- Altered tissue perfusion
- Impaired gas exchange
- Risk for altered body temperature
- Risk for perioperative positioning injury
- Pain
- Risk for impaired skin integrity

Interventions

Interventions are based on the nursing diagnoses. A plan of care will be designed to establish effective breathing and circulation, replace fluids, maintain body temperature, treat pain, prevent infection, promote effective elimination, and prevent intraoperative injury. Positioning is especially critical because the patient is at risk for a possible spinal fracture. A baseline neurological check is essential for determining disability before and after the surgical procedure. Postoperative care will focus on specific systems, as the goal is to identify actual and potential problems that may have occurred during surgery. The respiratory, cardiovascular, neurological, and renal systems and the surgical site are priorities for assessment and intervention.

Evaluation

Reflect upon the plan of care and readjust interventions according to patient needs.

Case Study: Mrs. W

A 78-year-old patient with Parkinson's disease fell at home and is admitted to the hospital with a diagnosis of intertrochanteric fracture of the left hip. The patient has had Parkinson's disease for several years and has been taking the medications Sinemet (carbidopa-levodopa) and Tasmar (tolcapone). What are the major concerns for this patient related to surgical intervention?

Points to Consider

- Health assessment, medical and surgical history.
- Major symptoms of Parkinson's disease.
- How will Parkinson's disease affect the patient's recovery and subsequent rehabilitation?
- What are the effects of the medications used to treat Parkinson's disease?
- Should particular attention be paid to intraoperative positioning for a patient with Parkinson's disease?
- Perioperative teaching.
- Discharge planning.

Case Study: Mr. R

A 55-year-old patient with a history of type I diabetes mellitus is scheduled for vascular surgery to restore and improve circulation to the right lower extremity. The patient has been on insulin therapy for several years and is knowledgeable about the disease but has problems complying with a routine schedule of testing blood glucose levels. In preparing this patient for surgery, what are important points for the perioperative nurse to consider in planning patient care?

Points to Consider

- Comprehensive health history and physical.
- Current blood glucose level and insulin therapy.
- Vascular assessment to include pulse, temperature, sensation, movement of lower extremities.
- Patient educational level.
- Nutritional assessment.
- Risk of impaired skin integrity and wound healing due to diabetes.
- Appropriate choice of fluid replacement.
- Level of impairment due to co-existing disease process.
- Neurological assessment.
- Relationship of NPO status to blood glucose levels and insulin therapy.
- Infection control measures.

Nursing Diagnoses

- Risk for infection
- Risk for impaired skin integrity
- Individual ineffective management of therapeutic regimen
- Altered tissue perfusion

Interventions are based on knowledge of the effects of the disease process (specifically diabetes mellitus) on the patient's course of care related to all body systems. Particular attention is paid to preventing infection and promoting wound healing.

Evaluation

Evaluation supports interventions and positive outcomes.

SUGGESTED LEARNING ACTIVITIES

- Review Perioperative texts (eg, *Alexander's Care of the Patient in Surgery, Berry & Kohn's Operating Room Technique, Care of the Patient During Operative and Invasive Procedures*) to increase your knowledge of optimizing physiologic protection; principles of positioning; and surgical, anesthetic, and perioperative interventions.

- Review anatomy and physiology texts.

- Review AORN's *Standards, Recommended Practices, and Guidelines* and the *Perioperative Nursing Data Set.*

- If you feel your patient assessment skills need improvement, seek out continuing education classes on assessment.

- Practice assessment with peers or family members. Choose various invasive procedures and plan the "patient's" care and your nursing interventions. Review these plans and interventions with peers and discuss your strengths and weaknesses.

- Evaluate your practice nursing care plans against this chapter's examples of how you can decrease the risk for physiological injury. For each sample "patient," evaluate how well you anticipated his or her risks and how effective your interventions were.

RECOMMENDED STUDY MATERIALS

AORN, *Standards, Recommended Practices, and Guidelines* (Denver: AORN, Inc, 2002).

Beyea, S, ed, *Perioperative Nursing Data Set,* second ed (Denver: AORN, Inc, 2002).

Phippen, M L; Wells, M P, *Patient Care During Operative and Invasive Procedures* (Philadelphia: W B Saunders Co, 2000).

Smeltzer, S; Bare, B, eds, *Brunner and Suddarth's Textbook of Medical-Surgical Nursing* (Philadelphia: Lippincott Williams and Wilkins, 2000).

CHAPTER 7: IMPLEMENT PLAN OF CARE TO ENHANCE PATIENT/ FAMILY EDUCATION

Susan Renée Guerra, RN, MN, CNOR, CNAA

This chapter provides the information necessary to conduct effective patient/family teaching. The effectiveness of nursing interventions is measured by patient outcomes. Teaching the patient and their support/family members about their surgical procedure, sequence of events in the perioperative process, and postoperative care can improve and ensure positive outcomes. The ultimate goal is to promote self-care and empower the patient to actively participate in each step of their surgical journey.

To ensure the teaching is appropriate, the desired outcomes must first be defined. Second, a thorough assessment of patient/family needs must be conducted on the following parameters: readiness to learn, cultural needs, language barriers, physiological status, psychological status, education level and experience, and the patient's values and wishes concerning care. The third step is to use this assessment information to develop a plan of care that identifies teaching methods and tools as well as timing and duration of teaching. Finally, teaching must be evaluated against the desired outcomes. Documentation of the teaching provided completes the legal requirements for education and allows fellow caregivers the opportunity to reinforce instruction.

LEARNING OBJECTIVES

1. Discuss assessment parameters that should be used to develop the teaching plan.

2. Identify expected outcomes of patient/family teaching.

3. Evaluate the effectiveness of teaching tools and methods according to established outcomes.

4. Describe various tools, media, and methods available to provide teaching.

5. Apply the principles of both child and adult learning to each teaching encounter.

TASK STATEMENT; AREAS OF KNOWLEDGE AND SKILL

Task Statement

Implement a plan of care to educate the patient/family to assist the patient in achieving optimal health status by using selected educational methods and resources. This also is accomplished by communicating information to minimize patient and family stress.

Areas of Knowledge

K-2 Anatomy and physiology
K-3 Pathophysiology
K-4 Pharmacology and anesthetic agents
K-5 Pain management
K-6 Principles of wound healing
K-7 Diagnostic procedures and results
K-8 Preoperative patient preparation activities
K-9 Surgical, anesthetic, and other perioperative interventions
K-10 Expected outcomes related to identified interventions
K-11 Physiologic responses to the surgical experience
K-13 Ergonomics and body mechanics
K-14 Transfer and transport techniques and equipment
K-17 Postoperative complications
K-20 Sociology (eg, cultural and ethnic influences, family patterns, spirituality and related practices)
K-21 Communication theories and techniques
K-22 Behavioral responses to the surgical experience
K-23 Discharge planning
K-24 Theories of and resources for patient/family education
K-25 *Perioperative Nursing Data Set* (PNDS)

K-27 Microbiology and infection control
K-28 Standard and transmission-based precautions
K-39 Patient rights and responsibilities
K-40 Legal responsibilities and implications for patient care
K-41 Approved nursing diagnoses (eg, NANDA)
K-42 Nursing research and evidence-based practice
K-43 "ANA Code of Ethics for Nurses with Explications for Perioperative Nurses"
K-44 Regulatory standards and voluntary guidelines
K-45 AORN *Standards, Recommended Practices, and Guidelines*
K-46 AORN position statements (eg, bloodborne pathogens, do-not-resuscitate orders [DNR])
K-47 Principles of problem solving
K-53 Quality improvement principles
K-49 Surgical consent laws and policies
K-50 Defining characteristics of impaired individuals (eg, substance abuse, psychological disturbance, compromised performance)
K-52 Defining characteristics of domestic abuse (eg, child, elder, partner/spouse)
K-54 Organ procurement
K-56 Implants (eg, handling, tracking, sterilization)

Areas of Skill

S-1 Confirming patient identity, operative site, and procedure
S-2 Collecting, analyzing, and prioritizing patient data
S-3 Using health assessment techniques (eg, interview, observation, auscultation, palpation, percussion)
S-4 Communicating effectively (verbal and nonverbal)
S-5 Advocating and protecting patient rights
S-6 Evaluating environment for discharge care
S-7 Assessing and managing pain
S-8 Assessing for potential abuse (eg, substance, domestic)
S-9 Assessing readiness to learn, knowledge level, and preferred learning style
S-10 Identifying barriers to learning
S-11 Identifying risk of infection and injury
S-12 Identifying cultural, spiritual, ethnic issues in care
S-13 Identifying age specific needs
S-14 Formulating a nursing diagnosis
S-15 Collaborating with other members on the health care team
S-16 Applying AORN *Standards, Recommended Practices, and Guidelines*
S-17 Applying the *Perioperative Nursing Data Set* (PNDS)
S-18 Delineating and communicating measurable patient outcomes
S-19 Participating in quality improvement activities
S-20 Maintaining accurate patient records
S-21 Protecting patients and members of the health care team from hazardous conditions
S-22 Providing evidence-based care
S-23 Applying regulatory standards and voluntary guidelines
S-24 Developing a patient and family education plan
S-25 Apply principles of and participate in cost containment, product evaluation, and resource management
S-26 Incorporating community and institutional resources into plan of care
S-27 Delegating interventions and/or assigning tasks
S-28 Adapting to changing situations and technologies
S-29 Performing nursing interventions
S-30 Documenting all relevant facts and data elements with appropriate terminology
S-35 Maintaining the dignity, modesty, and privacy of the patient and protecting the confidentiality of patient information
S-36 Applying principles of aseptic technique and infection control
S-43 Controlling environmental noise
S-44 Testing and using equipment
S-45 Monitoring physiological parameters
S-46 Anticipating and evaluating the effects of pharmacological and anesthetic agents
S-50 Adapting to special and unusual needs
S-52 Documenting nursing interventions and patient response
S-53 Educating, mentoring, and supervising health care team members
S-56 Measuring, evaluating, and documenting patient outcomes
S-61 Performing basic life support and other emergency procedures
S-62 Setting priorities
S-65 Applying ethical principles
S-67 Evaluating for signs and symptoms of injury
S-71 Securing patient belongings and valuables

DEVELOPING A PLAN OF CARE TO ENHANCE PATIENT/FAMILY EDUCATION

To develop a plan for patient/family education, each step in the process should be defined. This requires the perioperative nurse to identify the elements necessary to achieve the desired goals. The perioperative nurse must acquire an understanding of the surgical procedures and anesthesia techniques, age-specific learning principles, and teaching methods and available tools. The plan should be flexible to adapt to patient/family needs as well as many circumstances during which teaching may be performed.

The plan of care should incorporate the *Perioperative Nursing Data Set* (PNDS) vocabulary, which includes a section entitled "Behavioral Responses—Patient and Family: Knowledge." The PNDS language defines patient outcomes, outcome indicators, nursing interventions and activities, and evaluation methods necessary to ensure patient/family educational needs are met.

There are at least eight steps toward developing a patient/family education plan. Completion of each step will result in a comprehensive plan.

1. Define the patient assessment parameters.

Each patient must be thoroughly assessed before teaching is initiated. Information obtained during the patient assessment will allow the nurse to adapt the teaching plan to specific patient needs. Areas of assessment should include

- physiological status;
- psychosocial status;
- nutritional status and dietary preferences;
- allergies;
- education level;
- previous experience;
- readiness to learn;
- cultural needs;
- language requirements;
- substance abuse;
- expectations, personal needs, and requests,
- support systems;
- coping skills;
- home environment; and
- discharge planning needs.

2. List potential nursing diagnoses related to surgical procedure.

For each operative or invasive procedure, several nursing diagnoses should be identified. Actual and potential diagnoses should be cited so that the knowledge needs of each can be outlined. Nursing diagnoses for the disease process, surgical/invasive procedure, and knowledge needs can be addressed. Diagnoses specific to learning needs are

- deficient knowledge,
- anxiety,
- impaired home maintenance,
- ineffective coping,
- compromised family coping,
- decisional conflict, and
- body image disturbance.

3. Define the desired patient outcomes.

The best plans are developed with the end in mind. By defining the desired patient outcomes, the nurse can tailor the plan of care to ensure nursing interventions are performed to achieve the outcomes. The PNDS language uses six patient outcomes for patient knowledge.

- The patient demonstrates knowledge of the expected responses to the operative or other invasive procedure.
- The patient demonstrates knowledge of nutritional requirements related to the operative or other invasive procedure.
- The patient demonstrates knowledge of medication management.
- The patient demonstrates knowledge of pain management.
- The patient participates in the rehabilitation process.
- The patient demonstrates knowledge of wound management.

4. Identify the educational content required to address the knowledge needs of each nursing diagnosis and achieve each outcome.

Content designed to achieve each outcome can now be specified. This content should include, but not be limited to,

- preoperative preparation;
- operating room environment;
- basic anatomy and physiology related to the procedure;
- surgical procedure steps;
- anesthesia medications and techniques;
- sequence of events in the operating room;
- equipment used during the procedure;
- current patient medications and surgery medications—actions, indications, and side effects;
- pain management;
- postoperative wound care, including care of drains; and
- postoperative rehabilitation.

5. Outline teaching methods and tools available to provide the desired information.

The teaching methods and tools used will be determined by the patient assessment, available resources, skill of the nurse providing the education, the physical environment, and time available for instruction.

One to one—Most likely, the majority of the patient/family education will take place in one-to-one sessions. As much as possible, these should occur in areas without the potential for disruptions and in an environment that is conducive to learning. One-to-one teaching can be provided through each phase of the preoperative process.

Groups—These can be effective to provide information that is common across a number of surgical procedures. Groups also can be formed to provide information for patients preparing to undergo the same surgical procedure. Common information can include the operating room environment, anesthesia procedures, sequence of events, the postoperative recovery process, and pain control. Groups can provide the opportunity for patients and family members to learn from others through the comments made and questions asked.

Tours—Tours may be difficult to conduct due to ongoing patient activities and the need to maintain environmental control in restricted areas. If possible, patients and families can be shown where to go when they arrive at the facility for surgery. The postanesthesia care unit and next phase (ie, phase II) recovery are useful places for the patient and family members to tour; they can stimulate questions and discussion about the entire surgical process.

Questions and answers—The opportunity for the patient and family to ask questions should be used throughout the education process. This encourages the patient's and family members' involvement and can reinforce learning. It can provide an opportunity to the nurse to assess the effectiveness of the teaching.

Computer instruction—As the patient population becomes more computer savvy, computer instruction is a viable option to provide important information. Consistency of information is one advantage. Many programs allow the patient and family members to spend as much time as they need to absorb the instruction.

Videos—This media can be a great way to provide information to patients in a familiar format. When using videos, ensure that an overview of the content is provided before viewing so that the patient and family members know what they are expected to learn. At the end of the video, allow questions regarding the content and again review the key points.

Reading materials—Anxieties, disabilities, and many other factors can prevent verbal information from being absorbed. Any printed document that provides the information will be helpful. These can include pamphlets about the disease or surgical procedure, hospital information sheets, and written preoperative and postoperative instructions. The nurse must ensure that materials are provided in the patient's language.

Demonstration/return demonstration—Many activities can be shown to the patient and family members. Information is more likely to be retained if it can be reinforced through both words and actions. Actions such as coughing/deep breathing, log-rolling, and crutch walking lend themselves very well to this method.

Internet—Many resources are available on the Internet. Perioperative nurses must be cautious with this media, given that not all web sites provide current or accurate information. Patient and family members may be seeking information from this source, so it is a good idea for nurses to be prepared with some reputable web sites to provide to the patient. When possible, the nurse also can assess whether the patient/family has obtained information from this source so that the information can be reviewed and confirmed.

6. Identify where and when patient/family teaching will be performed.

Patient/family teaching can occur in a variety of settings and time frames and should not be restricted to any one location or structure. Teaching should be continuous throughout the perioperative process. Examples of appropriate teaching for each phase of the process are as follows.

Preoperative

- Provide verbal instruction.
- Provide instructions through written information, videos, and computerized instructions.
- Provide tours.

Intraoperative

- Provide reinforcement to preoperative teaching.
- Explain all procedures.
- Explain the purpose of specific equipment.
- Ensure conversation of room staff is appropriate at all times.
- Keep the family informed of the patient's condition and the progress of the procedure.

Postoperative

- Review the expected reaction to the surgery and

anesthesia.

- Encourage the patient to engage in self-care activities as much as possible.
- Reinforce pain management techniques.
- Encourage the family to support the process.
- Reinforce postoperative instructions, including diet, medications, activity limitations, and post-operative visits.
- Provide emergency contact information for the facility and the surgeon and identify those conditions that may alert an emergency.
- Connect the patient and family members to the discharge planner or long-term care assistance as indicated.

7. Define methods to evaluate effectiveness of patient/family learning.

To ensure the education provided is effective, the plan must include the method(s) used to evaluate learning.

Achievement of desired outcomes—Compare desired outcomes to actual outcomes to determine whether outcomes are met. Where not met, reassess the patient's needs and provide new instruction when appropriate.

Patient/family satisfaction—Satisfaction can be assessed by requesting verbal feedback from the patient and family. Formal satisfaction surveys can be provided at the point of discharge or sent to the patient and family after discharge.

Patient/family cognition—Determine if the patient and family members can verbalize an understanding of the teaching. Request the patient and family members to repeat the instructions that have been provided.

Patient/family psychomotor skills—Determine if the patient and family members are demonstrating the desired behaviors and can provide return demonstrations of specific activities.

Supportive resources—Assess whether family members or significant others demonstrate a willingness to be actively involved in the patient's care.

8. Identify where and how patient/family teaching will be documented.

Documentation of the education provided to the patient and family is an important final step in the plan of care. Careful documentation is important for many reasons, such as

- ensuring the patient and family receive a high standard of care,
- providing fellow caregivers with information about the education the patient and family have received so that teaching can be reinforced and enhanced,
- meeting regulatory requirements, and
- addressing legal concerns.

The plan should specify which forms will be used for documentation along with instructions for completing the forms. Forms should identify the information provided as well as the methods used. It is beneficial to have the patient and family members or other care provider sign that they have received the forms. All documentation must follow individual hospital policy.

IMPLEMENTING THE PLAN TO ENHANCE PATIENT/FAMILY EDUCATION

After developing the education plan outlined above, the perioperative nurse can implement the plan. The most effective implementation will be that which includes the principles of child and adult learning. The nurse must use the information obtained in the education assessment and apply it to ensure the appropriate learning principles are applied in each situation.

Principles of Child Learning and Development

- ◆ Children need to feel safe first.
  - Children develop and learn best where they are safe and valued, their physical needs are met, and they feel psychologically secure. Stress interferes with learning.

- ◆ Children learn through active engagement in their own learning.
  - Children know best how to go about learning something. If left alone, they will know instinctively what method is best for them. There is no need to motivate children through the use of extrinsic rewards, such as high grades or stars, which suggest to the child that the activity itself must be difficult or unpleasant (otherwise, why is a reward, which has nothing to do with the matter at hand, being offered?)

- ◆ Children are naturally curious.
  - Children want to make sense out of things, find out how things work, gain competence

and control over themselves and their environment, and do what they can see other people doing. They are open, perceptive, and experimental.

- Children learn through play.
  - Children learn through appropriate props, space, and time; and they become involved in the play by extending and elaborating on their ideas and language.
- Children need the opportunity to practice what they have learned.
  - Activities that allow for age appropriate demonstration and return demonstration are excellent to use with children.
- Provide the child with tasks he/she can accomplish.
  - Build on the child's strengths, celebrate what they can do, and encourage them to take risks. Give young children tasks that they can accomplish with effort, and present them with content that is accessible at their level of understanding.
- Children learn better in a supportive environment.
  - This principle of learning is that children can do things first in a supportive context and then later independently and in a variety of contexts.
- Children learn through repetition.
  - The child learner must start by repeating a limited amount of material many times over and over. Gradually, less and less repetition will be necessary to master new skills and new knowledge.

Principles of Adult Learning and Development

The learning principles for adults are similar in many ways, but differ in terms of building on current knowledge and experience. Malcolm Knowles was one of the first to describe the adult learning process. The principles he identifies below should be incorporated into the education approach for adults.

- Adults have a need to know why they should learn something. The adult has to consider it important to acquire the new skill knowledge or attitude.
- Adults have a need to be self-directing and decide for themselves what they want to learn.
- Adults have a far greater volume and different quality of experiences than young people, so connecting learning experiences to past experience(s) can make the learning experience more meaningful and help the participant acquire the new knowledge.
- Adults become ready to learn when they experience a life situation where they need to know.
- Adults enter into the learning process with a task centered orientation to learning.
- Adults are motivated to learn by both extrinsic and intrinsic motivation.

General Principles of Teaching

The nurse also must apply general principles of approaching both children and adults while teaching.

- Establish a rapport with both the patient and family.
- Use good communication skills using both verbal and nonverbal communication.
- Avoid a judgmental attitude.
- Communicate acceptance of the patient and family by projecting empathy and understanding and showing respect.
- Share the most important, relevant information first and cover only as much as the patient and family can assimilate during the time available.
- Encourage input and involvement in the teaching process.
- Create opportunities for patients and family members to participate in some activity.
- Involve as many senses as are appropriate for the situation—hearing, sight, feeling, and smell.
- Provide positive reinforcement to increase involvement and achievement of learning.
- Use the expertise of other health care professionals as necessary to address the short- and long-term learning needs.

SUMMARY

A comprehensive plan of care for patient/family teaching can help to ensure all desired patient outcomes are met. An effective teaching plan is one that includes a thorough assessment, identification of diagnoses, selection of appropriate teaching methods, and evaluation of learning. It is the responsibility of the perioperative nurse to implement the plan using an age-appropriate approach.

CASE STUDIES

Case Study: Mr. RW

Mr. RW is a retired 72-year-old male who is scheduled for a coronary artery bypass procedure. He has had two previous coronary arrests and has had two balloon angioplasties that were successful for a short period of time. During the last several years, RW has noticed that his hearing has become increasingly poor. He has difficulty distinguishing speech in noisy environments and relies on lip-reading when possible. He has refused to seek treatment for this and does not wear a hearing aid.

During the preoperative evaluation, you notice that he is alone. He frequently asks for information to be repeated. When asked a question, he responds with answers that do not reflect the question content. He fidgets with papers in front of him and does not seem to want the information about his procedure. While describing postoperative events and what will be expected of him, he waves his hand and says that he does not need to worry about that; the nurses will take care of him.

Points to Consider

- RW has many physiological problems that could affect his outcomes. What are his actual and potential physical limitations, and how can you include these in your teaching plan?
- He has arrived alone at the preoperative evaluation clinic. What specific assessment questions will you want to ask? What interdisciplinary team members might you consider consulting?
- Some of RW's nonverbal behavior provides clues to additional educational needs. Does he demonstrate readiness to learn? Does his behavior indicate anxiety?
- With RW's hearing deficit, how will you assess the effectiveness of the teaching you provide? How will you be certain he has been provided with all the appropriate information?

Discussion of Points to Consider

- Assessment
- Diagnoses
- Educational intervention
- Evaluation

Case Study: Ms. SB

SB is a 45-year-old female scheduled for an outpatient wide excision of a forearm skin lesion. She is attractive and appears confident. While completing your assessment, however, you discover that she is quite nervous about the procedure. She states that she is concerned she will have a large, visible scar on her forearm and that not all of her clothes will cover this. She also may have to have a skin graft from her thigh to cover a tissue deficit over the site. SB states the social circle in which she associates is very tuned in to physical appearance, and she fears she will not be as accepted in this group after the procedure.

The lesion itself could be malignant. She does not want to learn about the postoperative treatment should the lesion be cancerous, stating that she would face that later if she needed to. You notice she has a deep tan, and she confirm that she spends a great deal of time outdoors, either at the beach or playing tennis.

Points to Consider

- SB is displaying anxiety about the outcome of her surgery and voicing appropriate concerns about its immediate effects (ie, scarring, social acceptance). What approach can you take to lessen her anxiety?

- SB does not appear receptive to further information regarding the possibility of her lesion being cancerous. What can you do to promote her willingness to receive information about how to care for herself?

Discussion of Points to Consider

Education—Anxiety increases in situations in which the outcome is unknown. SB may have a significant knowledge deficit regarding her proposed surgery, thus her anxiety may be higher than normal. The nurse can discuss with her what she knows about the proposed procedure and correct any false impressions she may have. Showing the patient where the incision and graft site will be, discussing ways in which these areas may be camouflaged with clothing or makeup may be helpful. Education regarding how the body heals may be helpful in showing the patient that scars are not always as visible as they are initially and that they often become less noticeable over time may be helpful. This might also be a good time to introduce the effects of sun exposure on scar tissue and skin in general and help the patient see that she may need to take more precautions regarding tanning in the future.

Assessment and intervention—SB's ineffective coping with the possibility that her lesion may be cancerous and her anxiety about being accepted within her social circle can be eased somewhat by the use of open-ended, empathic statements such as "This must be hard for you to anticipate." These type of statements allow the patient to verbalize her fears and her plans for coping. Statements such as "The thought of a cancer diagnosis is scary. We can go over what you will need to do in that event postoperatively, if necessary," can allow the patient the time to assimilate the possibility of a cancer diagnosis and reassure her that you will be there to support her. Assessment of her social support system needs to be done to determine if a referral for counseling is appropriate.

Case Study: HC

HC is a 7-year-old female accompanied by her mother and 4-year-old sister to the day surgery unit. HC was born with a congenital foot defect that has required several surgeries. While checking the girl in for surgery, her mother burst into tears. She is a single mother who provides the support for both children. She has had to take the day off of work to be with her daughter for the procedure and is worried about her job. Child care for the sister and the patient after school has been difficult, causing the mother to have to leave work early on a regular basis. Her employer has stated she has until the end of the month to resolve the child care problems.

HC, as a veteran to the operating room, is very cooperative with all procedures but appears distressed about her mother. While the mother goes to the day surgery office to sign some papers, the patient expresses that she feels as if she is the cause of the problems. When asked if they have any other family members nearby, HC says that her grandparents live far away and she doesn't see them very often.

Points to Consider

- Children often feel as if they are responsible for family problems, and HC can see that she has some role in her mother's distress. She has felt safe enough to express her concerns and has apparently had positive experiences in the OR and learned to trust the nurses who care for her. How can you help this child feel more at ease regarding this difficult family situation?
- Parents, especially if they are single parents, are often emotionally stressed during a child's illness or surgery. HC's mother's ability to cope is impaired because of the additional stress of her work situation. This impairment can negatively affect and may prolong her child's recovery because of the inability to assimilate instructions and care requirements.

Discussion of Points to Consider

Assessment—Ask HC how she and her family have gotten through her past surgeries. Assess her social support system and what can be done to increase it. Discuss these issues with HC's mother and note the need for referral to counseling or other family support agencies.

Educational intervention—Reassure HC that she is not the cause of her mother's work problems and that it is natural for parents to be distressed when their children are sick or require surgery. Discuss with HC what she thinks would help her mother and her feel better. Remind HC that her surgeries are not indefinite and that soon she won't need further surgery on her foot. Review what to expect postoperatively and how she can participate in her care and speed her recovery. Let HC know that you will speak with her mother and help her mother find appropriate support personnel to help her through this surgery. Discuss postoperative care with HC's mother to evaluate how she has managed previously and what changes she could make. Provide the mother with support referrals as needed.

SUGGESTED LEARNING ACTIVITIES

Before implementing the education plan with actual patients, consider completing some or all of the following learning activities to develop and hone your skills.

- Select a specific surgical procedure and follow the steps to developing a complete education plan for that procedure.

- Identify specific and/or unique needs that you may encounter in your patient population. Using the assessment section of the education plan, state how you would adapt the plan to accommodate the specific needs.

- Prepare an inservice program for your peers that walks them through a patient/family education scenario from start to finish. Include the teaching that occurs during each of the perioperative phases. Describe how each staff member can maintain continuity of teaching and reinforce the teaching that has been provided.

- Schedule a meeting with the facility librarian and media specialist, if available. Ask these individuals to help identify additional resources and teaching tools that could be used for the perioperative population.

- Conduct an internet search to determine what information is available on specific surgical/invasive procedures. Confirm the currency and accuracy of content with your peers, interdisciplinary team members, and physicians.

- Develop a tool for documentation of education activities that incorporates each section of the teaching plan and ensures the PNDS language is used.

- Select a peer who is more experienced in patient/family teaching with whom you can practice a complete education plan. Request feedback on delivery, methods, and content.

- Contact company representatives who sell products and implants used for surgical procedures. Request they provide educational brochures, teaching guides, and sample products and implants that can be used for educational purposes.

RECOMMENDED STUDY MATERIALS

Abbott, S A, "The Benefits of Patient Education," *Gastroenterology Nursing* 21 (5) (September/October 1998) 207-209.

Abuksis, G; et al, "A Patient Education Program is Cost-Effective for Preventing Failure of Endoscopic Procedures in a Gastroenterology Department," *American Journal of Gastroenterology* 96 (6) (June 2001) 1786-90.

Adsit, K I, "Multimedia in Nursing and Patient Education," *Orthopedic Nursing* 15 (4) (July/August 1996) 59-63.

Ajam, M A, "Interactive Patient Education: The X-Plain Model," *Journal of Medical Practice Management* 16 (6) (May/June 2001) 301-305.

AORN, AORN's *Age-Specific Competencies Series* (Denver: AORN, Inc, 1997).

Beyea, S, ed, *Perioperative Nursing Data Set* second ed (Denver: AORN, Inc, 2002).

Best, J T, "Effective Teaching for the Elderly: Back to Basics," *Orthopedic Nursing* 20 (3) (May/June 2001) 46-52.

Bechtel, G A; Davidhizar, R E, "Integrating Cultural Diversity in Patient Education," *Seminars in Nursing Management* 7 (4) (December 1999) 193-197.

Brooks, B A, "Using the Internet for Patient Education," *Orthopedic Nursing* 20 (5) (September/October 2001) 69-77.

Byrne, M M, "Instructional Bias—Awareness and Reduction in Perioperative Education," *AORN Journal* 75 (4) (April 2002) 808-816.

D'Alfonso, J; Halvorson, C K, "E-learning in Perioperative Education," *SSM* 8 (2) (April 2002) 20-29.

Davidhizar, R; Bechtel, G; Dowd, S B, "Patient Education: A Mandate for Health Care in the 21st Century," *Journal of Nuclear Medicine Technology* 26 (4) (December 1998) 235-241.

Dreger, V; Tremback, T, "Optimize Patient Health by Treating Literacy and Language Barriers," *AORN Journal* 75 (2) (February 2002) 280-293.

Garity, J, "Cultural Competence in Patient Education," *Caring* 19 (3) (March 2000) 18-20.

"A Guide to Patient Education," *Orthopedic Nursing* 19 (Suppl) (May/June 2000) 5-9.

Hajewski, C, et al, "Implementation and Evaluation of Nursing Interventions Classification and Nursing Outcomes Classification in a Patient Education Plan," *Journal of Nursing Care Quality* 12 (5) (June 1998) 30-40.

"How to Document Patient Education Effectively," *Hospital Case Management* 7 (5) (May 1999) 94-95.

Knowles, M S, *The Modern Practice of Adult Education: Andragogy Versus Pedagogy* (New York: Association Press, 1970).

Leaffer, T; Gonda B, "The Internet: An Underutilized Tool in Patient Education," *Computers in Nursing* 18 (1) (January/February 2000) 47-52.

Maynard, A M, "Preparing Readable Patient Education Handouts," *Journal of Nurses Staff Development* 15 (1) (January/February 1999) 11-18.

Murphy, P W, et al, "Neurology Patient Education Materials: Do Our Educational Aids Fit Our Patients' Needs?" *Journal of Neuroscience Nursing* 33 (2) (April 2001) 99-104.

Palmerini, J; Jasovsky, D A, "Patient Education: A Guide for Success," *Nursing Management* 29 (9) (September 1998) 45-46.

Pittman, T J, et al, "Patient Education: Designing a State-of-the-Art Consumer Health Information Library," *Journal of Nursing Administration* 31 (6) (June 2002) 316-323.

Sanford, R C, "Caring Through Relation and Dialogue: A Nursing Perspective for Patient Education," *ANS: Advances in Nursing Science* 22 (3) (March 2000) 1-15.

Sasala, D B; Jasovsky, D A, "Using a Hospital-wide Performance Improvement Process for Patient Education Documentation," *Joint Commission Journal of Quality Improvement* 24 (6) (June 1998) 313-322.

Schrecengost, A, "Do Humorous Preoperative Teaching Strategies Work?" *AORN Journal* 74 (5) (November 2001) 683-689.

Shelswell, N L, "Perioperative Patient Education for Retinal Surgery," *AORN Journal* 75 (4) (April 2002) 801-807.

Ullrich, P R; Vaccaro, A R, "Patient Education on the Internet: Opportunities and Pitfalls," *Spine* 27 (7) (April 2002) 185-188.

Ward, S, et al, "Patient Education in Pain Control," *Support Care Cancer* 9 (3) (May 2001) 148-155.

Washburn, P V, "How to Improve Patient Education," *Hospital Topics* 78 (4) (Fall 2000) 5-8.

Watson, D S, "Education Programs in Surgical Services," *SSM* 8 (2) (April 2002) 16-19.

Williams, N H; Wolgin, F; Hodge, C S, "Creating and Educational Videotape," *Journal of Nurses Staff Development* 14 (6) (November/December 1998) 261-265.

Wood, B A, "Caring for a Limited-English Proficient Patient," *AORN Journal* 75 (2) (February 2002) 305-308.

Yellen, E; Davis, G C, "Patient Satisfaction in Ambulatory Surgery," *AORN Journal* 74 (4) (October 2001) 483-498.

CHAPTER 8: IMPLEMENT PLAN OF CARE CONSISTENT WITH PATIENT RIGHTS AND RESPONSIBILITIES

Cynthia K. Halvorson, RN, MSN, CNOR

The social context of health care has been undergoing several changes in the past few decades. Historically, the relationship between health care provider and patient was paternal in nature rather than a partnership. Two major factors have influenced this relationship and the perspective of the patient's involvement in his or her course of treatment.

First, an extraordinary revolution in the type, amount, and sources of information has increased the knowledge level of the patient. Internet-based information sources and direct-to-consumer marketing and promotion by pharmaceutical and medical technology companies are now common. Secondly, the focus of health care shifted from quality of care to efficiency and control of costs. Health insurance initiatives such as managed care and national health insurance have dramatically influenced the coordination, management, and financing of the system to combine the delivery and financing of health care. A part of these initiatives was an attempt to transform the patient into a consumer.

During the legislated and managed care initiatives, several statements or "bills" of patient rights have been put forth. Federal governmental efforts such as federal budget acts aimed to control cost and stipulate provider participation eligibility. Revisions of these acts include the right to grievance processes and freedom from nonmedically indicated restraints and seclusion. State legislative actions focused on provider liability and advanced directives. More recent legislation in the form of the Healthcare Insurance Portability and Accountability Act (HIPAA) addresses the right to sue the health plan provider, confidentiality of patient information contained within the medical record (particularly in automated, electronic format), and consent processes for access to the patient's health information for health care treatment, payment, and operations (TPO) as well non-TPO purposes.

Professional organizations such as the American Hospital Association (AHA), the American Medical Association (AMA), and the American Nurses Association (ANA) have established "bill of rights" and "code of ethics" for patient rights and provider conduct. The AHA Patients' Bill of Rights included statements of patient's rights to information and education; choice of treatment options, including refusal and privacy and confidentiality; access to medical records; patient information; and financial issues. The AMA and ANA documents include professional ethics in addition to patients' rights. Accreditation bodies such as the Joint Commission on Accreditation of Healthcare Organizations (JCAHO) have included patient rights and organization ethics in their standards of accreditation for health care facilities. Patients now expect and demand to be full and educated partners, making joint decisions with health care professionals.

Patients' rights and responsibilities are a complex mixture of legal and ethical principles. The core focus is toward optimal patient outcomes by ensuring the respect of each patient's basic rights in their health care and the provider's professional behavior and business conduct responsibilities.

Two main principles are patient autonomy and nonmaleficence. Autonomy is defined as the patient's self-determination or ability and power to make his or her own decisions regarding health care. Nonmaleficence involves acting in the best interest of the patient, for the benefit of patient. Justice or nonprejudicial care is provided for all patients regardless of values, culture, lifestyle, or economic considerations. These are incorporated into the individualized plan of care. Maintaining the confidentiality and privacy of related health information is defined as professional fidelity.

Both the ANA "Code of Ethics" and the AHA

"Bill of Rights" describe the role of professionals as patient advocate. Patient advocacy has two important functions: supporting the patient's autonomy and taking actions on behalf of the patient (beneficence) to ensure patient education, privacy, dignity, confidentiality, and safety.

The role of patient advocacy is central to perioperative nursing. The patient undergoing operative and invasive procedures has rights to determine their course of treatment. In addition, the patient is in a trust relationship, receiving a rapid sequence of care from a multidisciplinary team. Anesthesia administration, positioning requirements, and inherent risks of surgery require the perioperative nurse to be the patient advocate.

Examples of perioperative care in relation to patients' rights are

- patient identification and surgical site verification;
- supporting the patient in decision making;
- providing interpretative services for language barrier and hearing impairment needs;
- confirming informed consent (including adequate information, providing answers to questions, determining level of understanding);
- patient education regarding procedures, environment, and events;
- implementing advance directives policies;
- respecting patient decisions for advance directives and end of life choices;
- maintaining patient dignity with minimal exposure for prepping, draping, and other procedures (eg, foley catheter insertion) and keeping doors closed and windows covered;
- communicating with the health care team;
- refraining from discussing specific health information or aspects of the procedure in public areas; and
- verifying patient has appropriate transportation upon discharge.

LEARNING OBJECTIVES

1. Discuss the legal and ethical concepts related to patients' rights and responsibilities.
2. Discuss the organization's ethics and responsibilities in providing health care.
3. Explain patients' rights and responsibilities as they relate to access to care, informed consent, privacy and personal dignity, advanced directives, and patient charges.
4. List governmental agencies, accrediting bodies, and professional organization statements of patient rights.
5. Describe the perioperative nurse's role in ensuring patient rights and responsibilities are met.

TASK STATEMENT; AREAS OF KNOWLEDGE AND SKILL

Task Statement

Implement a plan of care that supports patients' rights, is consistent with clinical and legal standards, and includes patients in the decision-making process.

Areas of Knowledge

K-1 Health assessment techniques
K-4 Pharmacology and anesthetic agents
K-5 Pain management
K-10 Expected outcomes related to identified interventions
K-17 Postoperative complications
K-20 Sociology (eg, cultural and ethnic influences, family patterns, spirituality and related practices)
K-21 Communication theories and techniques
K-22 Behavioral responses to the surgical experience
K-23 Discharge planning
K-24 Theories of and resource for patient/family education
K-25 *Perioperative Nursing Data Set* (PNDS)
K-39 Patient rights and responsibilities
K-40 Legal responsibilities and implications for patient care
K-42 Nursing research and evidence-based practice
K-43 "ANA Code of Ethics for Nurses with Explications for Perioperative Nurses"
K-44 Regulatory standards and voluntary guidelines

K-45 AORN *Standards, Recommended Practices, and Guidelines*
K-46 AORN position statements (eg, bloodborne pathogens, do-not-resuscitate orders [DNR])
K-47 Principles of problem solving
K-49 Surgical consent laws and policies
K-52 Defining characteristics of domestic abuse (eg, child, elder, partner/spouse)
K-54 Organ procurement
K-55 Credentialing standards and clinical privileges
K-56 Implants (eg, handling, tracking, sterilization)

Areas of Skill

S-1 Confirming patient identity, operative site, and procedure
S-2 Collecting, analyzing, and prioritizing patient data
S-3 Using health assessment techniques (eg, interview, observation, auscultation, palpation, and percussion)
S-4 Communicating effectively (verbal and nonverbal)
S-5 Advocating and protecting patient rights
S-6 Evaluating environment for discharge care
S-7 Assessing and managing pain
S-8 Assessing for potential abuse (eg, substance, domestic)
S-9 Assessing readiness to learn, knowledge level, and preferred learning style
S-10 Identifying barriers to learning
S-11 Identifying risk of infection and injury
S-12 Identifying cultural, spiritual, and ethnic issues in care
S-13 Identifying age-specific needs
S-14 Formulating a nursing diagnosis
S-15 Collaborating with other members of the health care team
S-16 Applying AORN *Standards, Recommended Practices, and Guidelines*
S-17 Applying the *Perioperative Nursing Data Set* (PNDS)
S-18 Delineating and communicating measurable patient outcomes
S-20 Maintaining accurate patient records
S-21 Protecting patients and members of the health care team from hazardous conditions
S-22 Providing evidence based care
S-23 Applying regulatory standards and voluntary guidelines
S-24 Developing a patient and family education plan
S-25 Apply principles of and participate in cost containment, product evaluation, and resource management
S-26 Incorporating community and institutional resources into plan of care
S-27 Delegating interventions and/or assigning tasks
S-28 Adapting to changing situations and technologies
S-29 Performing nursing interventions
S-30 Documenting all relevant facts and data elements with appropriate terminology
S-35 Maintaining the dignity, modesty, and privacy of the patient and protecting the confidentiality of patient information
S-36 Applying principles of aseptic technique and infection control
S-49 Preparing and handling specimens for diagnostic evaluation
S-50 Adapting to special and unusual needs
S-51 Identifying and communicating changes in patient status
S-54 Recognizing impaired behavior in patients, family, and staff members and responding appropriately
S-55 Recognizing personal limitations and seeking assistance as needed
S-62 Setting priorities
S-63 Evaluating self and others according to goals and standards
S-64 Incorporating feedback into nurse performance
S-65 Applying ethical principles
S-66 Using resources for professional growth
S-69 Recording devices implanted or explanted during procedures
S-71 Securing patient belongings and valuables

PATIENT RIGHTS

Patient rights can be defined within several aspects of the health care experience.

- Patient Access to Care—Addresses patients' rights to fair and equal access to care and quality of care.
  - Reasonable access to care.
  - Care is provided fairly and equally; it is not based on nor denied because of national origin, sex, disability, color, race, religion, or source of payment.
  - Involved in all aspects of care.
  - Access to communication with visitors, through telephone calls and mail, unless treatment is compromised.
  - Access to interpretive services for those with a language barrier or hearing impairment.
  - Provided written statement of the institution's policy on patients' rights.

- Privacy and Personal Dignity—Addresses respect for basic human rights.
  - Treatment is with respect, dignity, and consideration.
  - Maintain personal privacy to extent possible during the course of treatment.
  - All communication and records pertaining to care is handled confidentially by only those providers directly involved in the patient's care.
  - Access to protective services such as guardianship, advocacy services, and child/adult protective services.
  - Access to pastoral care and counseling.
  - Resolution of complaints and conflict and ability to pursue grievances.

- Facility Staff Identification—Addresses the patient's right to know the identification, professional status, and competencies of the provider.
  - Knowledge of identity and professional status of care providers.
  - Each health care team member wears identification name badge.

- Informed—Addresses the patient's right to make own informed decisions based on information regarding treatment options, including the benefits, expected outcomes, and risks and potential complications; right to refuse treatment; and participation in research studies.
  - Involved in all aspects of care.
  - Informed about treatment.
  - Information about participation in investigational studies, clinical trials, and research, including expected benefits, potential risks and complications, alternative services, and full explanation of procedures to follow and comply; refusal to participate does not compromise access to service.
  - Family participates in care decisions.
  - Informed consent addresses expected outcomes/benefits, potential risks and complications, alternative treatment options, benefits and risks; potential outcome of refusal of treatment; name of person providing information; and date consent signed.
  - Informed of unanticipated outcomes.

- Advance Directives—Addresses the patient's right to indicate the decisions to be made and to authorize another to make decisions on his behalf if necessary.
  - Naming a substitute decision maker as permitted by law.
  - Formulation of advance directives (eg, living will) related to health care.

- Patient Charges—Addresses the patient's right to know the estimated cost of treatment and be provided with appropriate billing.
  - Ability to request, receive, and examine an itemized bill for services rendered in the facility.
  - Prior to the initiation of nonemergent treatment, upon request, right to be informed of routine, usual, and customary charges or estimate of charges for services.

- Patient Information and Confidentiality—Addresses the patient's right to protected health information including access and consent processes.
  - Access to medical record except as restricted by law.
  - Right to confidentiality of information.
  - Right to consent processes for treatment, payment, and care procedures as well as other requests for information.

- Additional Patient Rights
  - Option to transfer to another facility.
  - Option to consult with a specialist or to request a second opinion.
  - Assessment and management of pain.
  - Family members and primary care physician notified of admission.
  - Family involved in care decisions as appropriate.
  - Free of physical restraints or seclusion unless medically indicated.
  - Free of all forms of abuse and harassment.

PATIENT RESPONSIBILITIES

In addition to rights, patients also have responsibilities for participation in their care in order to ensure effective treatment and optimal outcomes.

- Providing Information
  - Providing accurate and complete information in matters related to their health, including present complaints, past illnesses, hospitalizations, and medications. Additionally, changes in health status and level of understanding must be communicated.

- Complying with Instructions
  - Following recommended treatment plan.
  - Asking questions and clarifications if directions and procedures are not understood.

- Informing the Practitioner of Refusal of Treatment
  - Informing the practitioner of refusal of treatment or noncompliance with treatment regimen.
  - Assuming responsibility for actions if treatment is refused.

- Following the Regulations of the Health Care Facility
  - Complying with facility's polices and regulations related to patients.
  - Consideration of other patients as well as facility personnel and property.

- Paying Health Care Facility Charges
  - Managing the financial obligations related to health care.

ORGANIZATIONAL ETHICS

Complementing the patient's rights and responsibilities are the facility's obligations and responsibilities under the law to operate with a code of ethical behavior.

- Marketing, admission, transfer and discharge, and billing practices are addressed.

- Clinical decision making is based on identified patient health care needs and not on use of services and financial incentives.

SUMMARY

A critical role of the perioperative nurse is advocacy for the surgical patient. The perioperative nurse is in a key position to ensure patients' rights and responsibilities and the organization's ethics in conducting business and professional behavior are met. Clinical decisions are made jointly by the patient and health care team. The patient's health care needs are matched to the facilities resources. Knowledge of practice standards, surgical procedures, and the health care facility's polices and regulations specific to patients' rights promote safe and effective care for optimal outcomes.

CASE STUDIES

Case Study: Dr. A

Ms. G is a specialty service manager at an urban teaching facility. Most of the team has been at the facility for several years. The specialty team and surgeons enjoy a very good working relationship. In appreciation, the surgeons host a social event twice a year for residents, fellows, and nursing staff members. Many of the perioperative staff members on the team consider the surgeons their friends. While in the service manager's office near the "control desk," Ms. G overheard one of her staff members discussing with several other staff members the urgent diagnostic procedure that Dr. A, one of the surgeons, had undergone over the weekend. The staff member related how she had entered the surgeon's computer medical records and how surprised she was at his age.

Points to Consider

- What violation of Dr. A's rights has occurred in this case study?

- How would you address the violation?

Discussion of Points to Consider

Dr. A's right to privacy and personal dignity and his right that all communication regarding his care be handled confidentially by only those providers directly involved in his care has been violated. Dr. A's privacy has been violated by the nurse overheard discussing his diagnostic procedure and information regarding his age that she retrieved from his medical record and has been discussing with other staff members.

It may be conceivable that this nurse is unaware of what she has done and by discussing what rights a patient is entitled to privately with her, you may have an opportunity to prevent further patient rights violations. If your private conversation is rebuffed and you feel that she will continue to discuss this information inappropriately, then a discussion with her supervisor of what you have overheard and your conversation with her may be necessary.

Case Study: Mrs. D

A 75-year-old Hispanic woman is scheduled for a laparoscopic cholecystectomy. She cannot read, speak, or understand English. Her 50-year-old son has accompanied her, but has limited English language skills. During the preoperative assessment, the perioperative nurse discovers a religious medallion taped to the patient's abdomen.

Points to Consider

- What patient rights have been compromised?
- How can you rectify what has occurred so far and see that this patient's care is not compromised in the future?

Discussion of Points to Consider

Patients have a right to interpretive services if there is a language barrier. Mrs. D cannot speak English, and her son apparently cannot speak or understand it fluently. This represents a severe compromise of Mrs. D's ability understand and participate in her care or to even consent to the care.

Mrs. D has a right to pastoral care and this care would probably help the nurse to understand the meaning of the religious medallion that had been taped to her abdomen. Clearly, its placement will interfere with her surgery, but it may be possible to have it placed elsewhere on her body and satisfy her need for its presence. A priest and an interpreter can discover this information and help soothe Mrs. D's anxieties about the impending surgery. By providing Mrs. D and her son with the interpreter and a priest, the nurse can rectify the problems that have occurred so far and improve their experience.

SUGGESTED LEARNING ACTIVITIES

- Review the American Nurses Association *Code of Ethics for Nurses with Interpretive Statements,* AORN's *Standards, Recommended Practices, and Guidelines,* and the *Perioperative Nursing Data Set.*
- Discuss with peers your institution's privacy policies and *The HIPAA Handbook: What Your Organization Should Know About the Federal Privacy Standards.*
- Discuss with peers patient care ethics.
- Explore what services your facility offers to aid patients and staff members (eg, interpreters, ethics boards or committees).

RECOMMENDED STUDY MATERIAL:

ANA, *Code of Ethics for Nurses with Interpretive Statements* (Washington, DC: American Nurses Association, 2001).

AORN, *Standards, Recommended Practices, and Guidelines* (Denver: AORN, Inc, 2002).

Berman S, "Setting Standards on Patient and Family Rights: An Interview with David Marx," *The Joint Commission Journal on Quality Improvement* 24 (11) (November 1999) 598-601.

Beyea, S, ed, *Perioperative Nursing Data Set,* second ed (Denver: AORN, Inc, 2002).

Brittin, A J; Melamed D, eds, *The HIPAA Handbook: What Your Organization Should Know About the Federal Privacy Standards* (Washington, DC, URAC/American Accreditation Healthcare Commission, 2001).

Byerly, R T; Carpenter E; Davis J, "Managed Care and the Evolution of Patient Rights," *JONA's Healthcare Law, Ethics, and Regulations* 3 (2) (June 2001) 58-67.

JCAHO, *2002 Hospital Accreditation Standards: Accreditation Polices, Standards, Intent Statements* (Oakbrook Terrace, Ill: Joint Commission on Accreditation of Healthcare Organizations, 2002).

Killen, A R; Fry S T; Damrosch S, "Ethics and Human Rights Issues in Perioperative Nurses: A Subsample of Maryland Nurses," *Seminars in Perioperative Nursing* 10 (4) (October 2001) 196-202.

Murphy, E K, "Preparation of the Patient for the Procedure: Legal and Ethical Considerations," in *Patient Care During Operative and Invasive Procedures,* Phippen, M L; Wells, M P, eds (Philadelphia: W B Saunders Co, 2000).

Rothman, D J, "The Origins and Consequences of Patient Autonomy: A 25-Year Retrospective," *Health Care Analysis* 9 (3) (2001) 255-254.

Schroeter, K, "Ethics in Perioperative Practice—Principles and Applications," *AORN Journal* 75 (4) (April 2002) 818-824.

Schroeter, K, "Ethics in Perioperative Practice—Patient Advocacy," *AORN Journal* 75 (5) (May 2002) 941-949.

CHAPTER 9: DOCUMENT PERIOPERATIVE ACTIVITIES

Janess Dulinski, RN, MSN, CNOR

Accurate documentation of patient status and patient care given is essential to perioperative nursing care. It is the surviving record of occurrences throughout the patient's surgical experience. Long after the room has been cleaned and the wound has healed, the patient's record will be the indicator of what happened while that patient was in our care.

The perioperative record serves as a communication tool among colleagues. Verbal report is given between nurses as the patient is delivered into the care of the next specialist. Written documentation allows reference back to information shared.

It is essential that the information that is documented be accurate and that time is taken with the patient to extract details that may be forgotten in a time of stress, such as the perioperative experience. Surgery often occurs within an hour or two of the patient entering the institution; patients often are discharged before the end of the day. Therefore, accurate, timely, up-to-date documentation is crucial.

This chapter discusses the documentation of the perioperative experience. Emphasis is placed on intraoperative documentation, while addressing preoperative and immediate postoperative concerns.

LEARNING OBJECTIVES

1. Delineate the elements of perioperative documentation.

2. Discuss the rationale of accurate and complete patient assessment and perioperative nursing activities.

3. Participate in institutional perioperative nursing documentation formats.

TASK STATEMENT; AREAS OF KNOWLEDGE AND SKILL

Task Statement

Document perioperative nursing practice to provide a permanent record for continuity of patient care, quality improvement, and accountability. This is accomplished by recording observations, nursing activities, patient responses, and other relevant data.

Areas of Knowledge

K-1 Health assessment techniques
K-2 Anatomy and physiology
K-3 Pathophysiology
K-4 Pharmacology and anesthetic agents
K-5 Pain management
K-6 Principles of wound healing
K-7 Diagnostic procedures and results
K-8 Preoperative patient preparation activities
K-9 Surgical, anesthetic, and other perioperative interventions
K-10 Expected outcomes related to identified interventions
K-11 Physiologic responses to the surgical experience
K-12 Principles of positioning
K-14 Transfer and transport techniques and equipment
K-15 Risks for injury, including but not limited to, skin, positioning, and retained foreign body
K-16 Emergency procedures (eg, CPR, MH)
K-17 Postoperative complications
K-18 Defining characteristics of impending patient physiologic crisis
K-19 Emergency operative procedures
K-20 Sociology (eg, cultural and ethnic influences, family patterns, spirituality and related practices)
K-21 Communication theories and techniques

K-22 Behavioral responses to the surgical experience
K-23 Discharge planning
K-24 Theories of and resources for patient/family education
K-25 *Perioperative Nursing Data Set* (PNDS)
K-26 Requirements for handling of specimens
K-27 Microbiology and infection control
K-28 Standard and transmission-based precautions
K-29 Potential hazards in the perioperative environment including, but not limited to, chemical, electrical, fire, gas, laser, physical environment, radiologic, extraneous objects
K-30 Interventions to optimize safety
K-31 Technologies and equipment relating to perioperative practice
K-32 Environmental parameters (eg, temperature, humidity, air exchange)
K-33 Principles of sterilization and disinfection
K-34 Protective barrier materials
K-37 Principles of product evaluation, cost-containment and resource management
K-39 Patient rights and responsibilities
K-40 Legal responsibilities and implications for patient care
K-41 Approved nursing diagnoses (eg, NANDA)
K-42 Nursing research and evidence-based practice
K-44 Regulatory standards and voluntary guidelines
K-45 AORN *Standards, Recommended Practices, and Guidelines*
K-46 AORN position statements (eg, bloodborne pathogens, do-not-resuscitate [DNR] orders)
K-47 Principles of problem solving
K-48 Quality improvement principles
K-49 Surgical consent laws and policies
K-50 Defining characteristics of impaired individuals (eg, substance abuse, psychological disturbance, compromised performance)
K-52 Defining characteristics of domestic abuse (eg, child, elder, partner/spouse)
K-54 Organ procurement
K-55 Credentialing standards and clinical privileges
K-56 Implants (eg, handling, tracking, sterilization)

Areas of Skill

S-1 Confirming patient identity, operative site, and procedure
S-2 Collecting, analyzing, and prioritizing patient data
S-3 Using health assessment techniques (eg, interview, observation, auscultation, palpation, percussion)
S-4 Communicating effectively (verbal and nonverbal)
S-5 Advocating and protecting patient rights
S-6 Evaluating environment for discharge care
S-7 Assessing and managing pain
S-8 Assessing for potential abuse (eg, substance, domestic)
S-10 Identifying barriers to learning
S-11 Identifying risk of infection and injury
S-12 Identifying cultural, spiritual, ethnic issues in care
S-13 Identifying age specific needs
S-14 Formulating a nursing diagnosis
S-16 Applying AORN *Standards, Recommended Practices, and Guidelines*
S-17 Applying the *Perioperative Nursing Data Set* (PNDS)
S-18 Delineating and communicating measurable patient outcomes
S-19 Participating in quality improvement activities
S-20 Maintaining accurate patient records
S-22 Providing evidence-based care
S-23 Applying regulatory standards and voluntary guidelines
S-24 Developing a patient and family education plan
S-26 Incorporating community and institutional resources into plan of care
S-28 Adapting to changing situations and technologies
S-30 Documenting all relevant facts and data elements with appropriate terminology
S-31 Recording unusual occurrences and/or variances in care
S-35 Maintaining the dignity, modesty, and privacy of the patient and protecting the confidentiality of patient information
S-46 Anticipating and evaluating the effects of pharmacological and anesthetic agents
S-47 Documenting maintenance of a safe environment
S-49 Preparing and handling specimens for diagnostic evaluation
S-51 Identifying and communicating changes in patient status
S-52 Documenting nursing interventions and patient response
S-56 Measuring, evaluating, and documenting patient outcomes
S-65 Applying ethical principles
S-67 Evaluating for signs and symptoms of injury
S-68 Performing required counts
S-69 Recording devices implanted or explanted during procedures
S-70 Classifying the surgical wound
S-71 Securing patient belongings and valuables

RATIONALE FOR DOCUMENTATION

Documentation serves as a written record of perioperative nursing care including patient assessment, the actions taken as a result of that assessment, the plan of care developed and implemented, and the results of all of these actions. Documentation serves as a communication tool for the health care team and as a means of improving care through retrospective studies. As stated in AORN's 2002 *Standards, Recommended Practices, and Guidelines,* "Perioperative documentation is essential for the continuity of goal-directed care and for comparing achieved patient outcomes to expected patient outcomes."

DOCUMENTATION METHODS

A variety of methods may be used for the documentation of perioperative care. Health care facilities will most often require the use of one standard method throughout the institution. Standardization enables staff members to retrieve information in a timely manner.

The perioperative nurse is encouraged to participate in the decision making process when the institution reviews documentation methods. The perioperative nurse has an insight to the requirements for this specialty area. The CNOR candidate should be familiar with the *Perioperative Nursing Data Set* (PNDS) as developed by AORN. The CNOR serves as leader by example and should guide others toward the utilization of this most useful tool for continuity in nursing documentation.

Some common methods for documentation of nursing activities include

- SOAP—subjective, objective, analysis, and planning;
- APIE—assessment, planning, implementation, evaluation;
- POMR—problem-oriented medical record; and
- source oriented recording—chronology of patient care and assessment.

The above listed methods can be time consuming and often do not address the assessment and the actions taken on behalf of the perioperative patient. Most surgical facilities have therefore created a form or forms that address this unique situation. The perioperative nurse is encouraged to participate in the development and revision of such forms. As information technology increases throughout health care institutions, the perioperative nurse needs to be familiar with various programs and be involved in the use of this means of documentation.

TYPES OF FORMS USED FOR DOCUMENTATION

The form or forms developed by the institution will address the needs of the patients in the particular environment. Whether the documentation is a fold-out continuum or a collection of area-specific forms, the following will need to be addressed and made available to everyone caring for patients.

Nursing Interview Form

This form may be a generalized form, for medical and surgical patients alike. This form addresses reason for hospitalization, activities of daily living, language barriers, psychosocial history, advance directive status, plans for discharge, and postdischarge care. It should be specific to nursing and not duplicate the medical history.

Preoperative Assessment Form/Checklist

This form is specific for the patient experiencing an invasive procedure. It addresses areas of concern specific to the operative patient. Information noted may include, but is not limited to, the following.

- Patient identification and allergy bracelet in place.
- Medical/surgical history—listing of pre-existing conditions that will affect the care given this patient. Patient history addressed here will be incorporated into the nursing care plan.
- Physical limitations—sensorial and mobility limitations need to be listed and addressed in the nursing care plan. Location of sensory aids and/or prosthetics need to be documented.
- Presence of operative consent with verification of site of surgery—the nurse documents the presence of the consent and any concerns the patient expresses regarding the procedure. The surgeon needs to be notified of any patient concerns. This notification also needs to be documented.
- Preoperative teaching—this will be incorporated into the nursing care plan

- Location of family members during the procedure.
- Allergies—this vital information must be obvious to all caring for patients.
- NPO status—especially important for general anesthesia candidates.
- Level of consciousness and emotional status—provides a baseline for later assessments.
- Patient height, weight, and vital signs—allows for accurate medication dosing and provides a baseline for later assessments.
- Presence of physician's history and physical.
- Presence of laboratory tests and imaging.
- Preoperative medications.
- Blood products given and availability—essential in some situations.

Intraoperative Form/Checklist

The information commonly noted here will be discussed in the Intraoperative Nursing Activities section.

Postoperative Assessment

This form is used by the postanesthesia care provider.

DOCUMENTATION OF PLAN OF CARE

A plan of care for the patient is required by the Joint Commission on Accreditation of Healthcare Organizations (JCAHO) and needs to be in the patient's record before any procedure is performed. The plan must be individualized and current. As the condition of the patient varies, the plan must be adjusted to meet the current needs of the patient.

The plan includes the following:

- nursing plan of care;
- plan for the operative or other procedure;
- a postprocedure plan of care;
- assessment of the need for additional diagnostic data;
- assessment of the patient's acuity to determine the appropriate level of post-procedure care; and
- assessment of the patient's physical, mental, and neurological status.

These plans of care are often incorporated into the perioperative nursing documentation form(s).

INTRAOPERATIVE NURSING ACTIVITIES

Documentation of direct patient care during the intraoperative phase should reflect evidence of continued assessment, adaptation, and adjustment of the nursing care provided. The perioperative nurse reviews the preoperative assessment and verifies the information listed. Intraoperative documentation should include, but not be limited to,

- site of surgery verification;
- patient position—placement of limbs, positioning devices used, padding used;
- safety device placement—lead shielding, safety straps, electrocautery dispersive electrode (ie, patient ground);
- location of monitoring devices;
- skin condition—color, turgor, temperature;
- equipment used, along with settings;
- operative times, including patient entry and discharge from the OR suite, anesthesia start and finish, surgical start and finish;
- procedure performed;
- preoperative and postoperative diagnosis;
- complications, if any;
- people present for procedure (eg, surgeon, assistants, anesthesia care providers, nursing staff [including changes of staff with times], technical staff [x-ray technicians, perfusionists, other monitoring staff], industry partners, and student observers when permitted);
- skin prep—shave and solutions used;
- catheters placed—urine output prn;

- disposition of specimens;
- wound classification;
- irrigation used;
- medications administered;
- implants and explants;
- closure method;
- dressing applied;
- transportation method;
- level of consciousness;
- airway status; and
- transport accessories (eg, monitors, oxygen).

POSTOPERATIVE NURSING ACTIVITIES

Postoperative nursing activities, whether performed in the postanesthesia care unit or in the ambulatory surgery recovery area (in the case of local anesthesia) are often incorporated into the continuum of the perioperative documentation. Appropriate notation of this aspect of patient care is addressed by the postanesthesia care nurse colleague.

SUMMARY

Perioperative documentation is an essential portion of the nursing care given. Without a lasting form of communication among caregivers, vital patient data may be forgotten or overlooked, breaking the continuum of care. Review, at the time of need, of written documentation provides assurance of assessment made and previous care given, along with providing a base for planning of care to be given.

Nursing, as a profession, must plan its own care. The nurse plans the improvement of care given by developing a documentation format. The format is used by the nurse caregiver. Periodic assessment of the documentation, by use of retrospective studies and chart reviews, allows the nursing team to determine the effectiveness of the format. By using the nursing process, nursing continues to improve patient care. The perioperative nurse, through dedication to the perioperative patient, study, and involvement in continuous quality improvement, positively affects the care given to surgical patients.

CASE STUDIES

Specific issues will be addressed and emphasized in the following case studies. Common perioperative assessment and documentation will be understood as carried out.

Case Study: Ms. B

Preoperative

Ms. B is brought to surgery for a right breast biopsy under local anesthesia. Ms. B is 45 years old and the mother of two young boys. During the preoperative assessment, the nurse is told that Ms. B's mother died of breast cancer. The patient denies allergies to medications, but indicates she once experienced a prolonged irritation when she applied iodine to a cut. Vital signs are taken and are within normal parameters.

Documentation:

- The perioperative nurse documents the close family history of breast cancer.
- Plan of care includes emotional support of patient throughout surgical experience.
- The nurse documents the potential allergy to iodine-based products.
- Plan of care includes use of an alternative surgical prep solution.
- The nurse documents the location of surgery per patient interview and verifies the correctness of the consent.

Intraoperative

Ms. B is brought to the OR and again asked as to the nature and the location of the procedure to be performed. The consent is reviewed, and the surgeon verifies the site. The nurse, serving as the monitoring nurse, applies electrodes and other monitoring devices. The initial intraoperative vital signs are taken. Preoperative assessment documented potential allergy to iodine. An alternative prepping solution is chosen. The surgeon administers lidocaine 1% with epinephrine 1:100,00. As the surgery proceeds, the monitoring nurse takes vital signs on a regular basis, checks the patient's perception of pain, and remains alert for indications of adverse reaction to the local anesthetic agent. The specimen is sent fresh to pathology. The wound is closed with a subcuticular closure and steristrips. A light dressing is applied.

Documentation:

- The nurse documents verification of surgical site.

- The monitoring nurses documents location of monitoring devices, periodic vital signs, patient perception of pain, and any indication of adverse reaction.
- The nurse documents the prep solution used.
- The nurse documents the specimen, including description, destination, and requested diagnostic procedure.

Postoperative

The perioperative nurse assesses the surgical site for skin integrity. The monitoring nurse calls the ambulatory surgery area to alert them to the return of the patient and to give a verbal report on the condition of the patient. The patient is returned to the ambulatory surgery area.

Documentation:

- Plan of care continues with assessment of the results of nursing care.

Case Study: Ms. H

Preoperative

Ms. H has been hospitalized with a left intertrochanteric hip fracture. It is determined that this patient needs surgery and is scheduled for a left hip pinning. Ms. H is 82 years old and lives alone in an apartment. She has a daughter who lives about a mile away and visits Ms. H often. Ms. H is active with her church. She broke her hip while boarding a bus with her church group to spend a day at a museum. The patient is 5 ft tall and weighed 96 lbs. when she visited her doctor last month. She denies allergies to medications. Vital signs and lab work are within normal parameters. Hematocrit is 37%, and hemoglobin is 12 g/dl on admission.

Documentation:

- The perioperative nurse documents the patient's orientation.
- Plan of care includes patient education and inclusion of the patient in all care decisions to meet this patient's age-specific needs.
- The nurse documents the blood values as being on the low side of normal.
- Plan of care includes inquiring as to the potential need for blood product availability.
- The nurse documents the location of surgery per patient interview and verifies the correctness of the consent.

Intraoperative

Ms. H is brought to the OR and again asked as to the nature and location of the procedure to be performed. The consent is reviewed. The blood bank is called to confirm the availability of two units of packed red blood cells. Location of the patient's blood band and identification number are noted. A spinal anesthesia is administered. The patient is transferred to the fracture table and placed in bilateral traction. Given the age and size of the patient, care is given to padding bony prominences and careful abduction of the legs. The left arm is padded and positioned across the chest. The right arm is secured on a padded arm board. A forced-air warming blanket is applied, and the patient is prepped and draped. The surgery proceeds smoothly. A lag screw with 4-hole side plate are used to reduce and secure the fracture. A closed wound suction drain is placed in the wound as it is closed. A medium dressing is applied.

Documentation:

- The nurse documents verification of the surgical site.
- The nurse documents the location and individual identification number of the patient's blood band.
- The nurse documents positioning and padding actions taken to protect the patient.
- The nurse documents the nature, location, size, lot numbers, and expiration dates (if any) of all implants.
- The nurse documents the nature, location, and size of the drain used.

Postoperative

The patient is transferred to the transport cart. Skin is assessed for evidence of pressure damage. The patient is transported to the postanesthesia care unit with oxygen per mask.

- The nurse documents skin integrity.
- The nurse documents transport destination, means (eg, cart, bed) and transport accessories (oxygen per mask).

SUGGESTED LEARNING ACTIVITIES

Throughout your career, periodically audit your own documentation. As a certified perioperative nurse, you lead by example. In preparation for your certification exam, you may find it helpful to consider one or more of the following activities.

- ◆ Choose a colleague you respect for the care given

and suggest auditing each other's documentation. Periodically obtain records of patients from the medical records department. Discuss findings and offer suggestions for improvement.

- Meet with your institution's risk management team. Review documentation requirements.
- Prepare an in-service program for your department to discuss appropriate documentation of perioperative care. Work with your colleagues to identify variances of form completion; strive for continuity.

RECOMMENDED STUDY MATERIALS

AORN, "Recommended Practices for Documentation of Perioperative Nursing Care," in *Standards, Recommended Practices, and Guidelines* (Denver: AORN, Inc, 2002).

Beyea, S C, "The Ideal State for Perioperative Nursing," *AORN Journal* 73 (5) (2001) 897-901.

Fortunato, N H, ed, *Berry & Kohn's Operating Room Technique*, ninth ed (St Louis: Mosby, Inc, 2000).

Fairchild, S S, *Perioperative Nursing, Principles and Practice* (Boston: Little, Brown and Co, 1996).

Gruendemann, B J; Fernsebner, B, *Comprehensive Perioperative Nursing* Vol 1 (Boston: Jones and Bartlett, 1995).

JCAHO, *2002 Hospital Accreditation Standards: Accreditation Polices, Standards, Intent Statements* (Oakbrook Terrace, Ill: Joint Commission on Accreditation of Healthcare Organizations, 2002).

Meeker, M H; Rothrock, J C, *Alexander's Care of the Patient in Surgery,* 12th ed (St Louis: Mosby, Inc, 2002).

CHAPTER 10: EVALUATE PATIENT RESPONSE TO PLAN OF CARE

Linda K. Groah, RN, MS, CNOR, CNAA, FAAN

The final step in the nursing process is evaluating the effectiveness of the nursing activities that have been implemented. Evaluation involves collecting data that identifies the effects of nursing interventions, then comparing that data to predefined outcome criteria to measure whether the desired outcomes for the patient have been met. The result of this process is to provide information that allows the nurse to modify the plan of care at any stage in the patient's perioperative experience.

The evaluation component also is applied to the assessment and implementation of plans that are used to improve systems and services required for safe, effective patient care delivery. This increases the potential of achieving the desired outcomes for all perioperative patients.

Under the supervision of the perioperative nurse, properly trained, unlicensed assistive personnel may collect data that can be used in the evaluation of patient response to care. However, the critical thinking and nursing judgment required to determine the effectiveness of the care that is delivered, and any modifications to the plan, requires the education and knowledge of the registered nurse in the perioperative setting.

This chapter provides the nurse with information related to evaluating the effectiveness of services and of the nursing interventions identified in the plan of care and provided to the patient. This requires that the nurse be able to

- identify expected patient outcomes and write criteria that are used to measure those outcomes;
- collect and interpret data from patient responses that can be used to judge whether criteria have been met;
- analyze evaluation data to determine what additions or modifications to the plan of care may be appropriate;
- communicate this information both verbally and in writing in a meaningful manner to other members of the health care team; and
- determine the effectiveness of nursing care provided to meet the desired patient outcomes.

This chapter reviews the areas of knowledge and skill that are used in evaluating nursing interventions in the preoperative, intraoperative, and postoperative periods. Nurses will have the opportunity to identify their learning needs related to evaluation by responding to questions based on the case studies provided. In addition, nurses will enhance their skills in this area by performing the learning activities suggested in this section. The chapter concludes with a bibliographical listing of the recommended study materials.

LEARNING OBJECTIVES

Individuals preparing for the CNOR exam should direct their study activities toward obtaining the specific areas of knowledge and skill required for evaluating patient responses to nursing interventions. When the content of this chapter has been completed, the nurse will be able to:

1. Write specific and individualized criteria that may be used in the measurement of patient outcomes.
2. Collect data in a manner that allows for consistent measurement of responses by any health care team member involved in the evaluation process.
3. Analyze data collected to determine if outcome

criteria have been met.

4. Identify further nursing actions that are necessary, based on the degree to which the patient outcomes were achieved.

5. Communicate the status of patient outcome attainment.

6. Evaluate the quality of nursing care and services provided to the patient.

TASK STATEMENT; AREAS OF KNOWLEDGE AND SKILL

Task Statement

Evaluate patient response to the plan of care by determining the achievement of expected outcomes by continuously assessing the health status of the patient.

Areas of Knowledge

K-1 Health assessment techniques
K-2 Anatomy and physiology
K-3 Pathophysiology
K-4 Pharmacology and anesthetic agents
K-5 Pain management
K-6 Principles of wound healing
K-7 Diagnostic procedures and results
K-8 Preoperative patient preparation activities
K-9 Surgical, anesthetic, and other perioperative interventions
K-10 Expected outcomes related to identified interventions
K-11 Physiologic responses to the surgical experience
K-15 Risks for injury, including but not limited to skin, positioning, and retained foreign body
K-17 Postoperative complications
K-18 Defining characteristics of impending patient physiologic crisis
K-20 Sociology (eg, cultural and ethnic influences, family patterns, spirituality and related practices)
K-21 Communication theories and techniques
K-22 Behavioral responses to the surgical experience
K-23 Discharge planning
K-24 Theories of and resources for patient/family education
K-25 *Perioperative Nursing Data Set* (PNDS)
K-27 Microbiology and infection control
K-28 Standard and transmission-based precautions
K-31 Technologies and equipment relating to perioperative practice
K-32 Environmental parameters (eg, temperature, humidity, air exchange)
K-39 Patient rights and responsibilities
K-40 Legal responsibilities and implications for patient care
K-41 Approved nursing diagnoses (eg, NANDA)
K-42 Nursing research and evidence-based practice
K-43 "ANA Code of Ethics for Nurses with Explications for Perioperative Nurses"
K-44 Regulatory standards and voluntary guidelines
K-45 AORN *Standards, Recommended Practices, and Guidelines*
K-46 AORN position statements (eg, bloodborne pathogens, do-not-resuscitate orders [DNR])
K-47 Principles of problem solving
K-50 Defining characteristics of impaired individuals (eg, substance abuse, psychological disturbance, compromised performance)
K-52 Defining characteristics of domestic abuse (eg, child, elder, partner/spouse)
K-56 Implants (eg, handling, tracking, sterilization)

Areas of Skill

S-1 Confirming patient identity, operative site, and procedure
S-2 Collecting, analyzing, and prioritizing patient data
S-3 Using health assessment techniques (eg, interview, observation, auscultation, palpation, percussion)
S-4 Communicating effectively (verbal and nonverbal)
S-5 Advocating and protecting patient rights
S-7 Assessing and managing pain
S-8 Assessing for potential abuse (eg, substance, domestic)
S-9 Assessing readiness to learn, knowledge level, and preferred learning style
S-10 Identifying barriers to learning
S-11 Identifying risk of infection and injury
S-12 Identifying cultural, spiritual, ethnic issues in care
S-13 Identifying age specific needs
S-15 Collaborating with other members on the health care team
S-16 Applying AORN *Standards, Recommended Practices, and Guidelines*
S-17 Applying the *Perioperative Nursing Data Set* (PNDS)
S-18 Delineating and communicating measurable patient outcomes
S-19 Participating in quality improvement activities
S-20 Maintaining accurate patient records
S-22 Providing evidence based care

S-23 Applying regulatory standards and voluntary guidelines
S-27 Delegating interventions and/or assigning tasks
S-28 Adapting to changing situations and technologies
S-30 Documenting all relevant facts and data elements with appropriate terminology
S-31 Recording unusual occurrences and/or variances in care
S-35 Maintaining the dignity, modesty, and privacy of the patient and protecting the confidentiality of patient information
S-45 Monitoring physiological parameters
S-46 Anticipating and evaluating the effects of pharmacological and anesthetic agents
S-50 Adapting to special and unusual needs
S-51 Identifying and communicating changes in patient status
S-52 Documenting nursing interventions and patient response
S-56 Measuring, evaluating, and documenting patient outcomes
S-65 Applying ethical principles
S-67 Evaluating for signs and symptoms of injury

PREOPERATIVE NURSING ACTIVITIES

After the initial assessment is completed, the next step in the nursing process is to use the assessment data to establish nursing diagnoses. The perioperative nurse then identifies expected patient outcomes and develops a plan of care to help the patient achieve those outcomes, thus establishing a framework for later evaluation of nursing care.

An outcome standard or goal establishes an essential condition or limitation that is necessary for safe nursing care. For example, it is important for patients to know about their medications before discharge. If the outcome states, "Patient knows the side effects of medications," the nurse has a responsibility to instruct the patient and to evaluate his or her knowledge of those side effects.

Of all the various types of patient care standards, outcome standards are the most practical and the easiest to develop and measure. This is because nurses are using most of the outcomes included in these standards in their plans of care. Although nurses may differ in the actions that they use to achieve the desired result, the outcome criteria for these standards should only specify patient behaviors that result from the delivery of appropriate and competent nursing care.

Patient outcome standards should address the following areas:

◆ Routine but high-risk/high-incident problem areas that are applicable to the care of any surgical patient
  - Standards 1.1 to 1.9 of AORN's "Patient Outcomes: Standards for Perioperative Care" have established outcomes for the high-risk/high-incident problem areas.

◆ Problem areas specific to the individual patient
  - These problem areas are derived from the assessment data collected specifically for each patient.

Based on these patient outcome standards, the evaluation process includes the following.

◆ Development of outcome criteria

Outcome criteria are developed to identify the tasks or conditions to be implemented that will assist the patient in achieving the desired outcomes. These criteria serve as a "checklist" against which to compare the patient's actual condition after the plan has been implemented. Outcome criteria indicate an expected, measurable change in the patient's health status. Patient outcomes are probably the most important indicators of the quality of the nursing care that has been provided.

Outcome criteria may include any of the following indicators:
- Expected physiological signs and symptoms
- Expected psychological and emotional status
- Behavioral expectations
- Results from laboratory or diagnostic tests
- Patient statements

An example of a patient outcome for the preoperative period and its related outcome criteria follows.
- Expected Outcome: The patient demonstrates knowledge of the physiological and psychological responses to surgical intervention.
- Outcome Criteria: The patient will be able to:
  a. Describe the surgical procedure to be performed in his own words
  b. Ask questions related to the perioperative care to be provided
  c. Interpret his understanding of the care to

be provided

d. State concerns related to the surgical procedure
e. State outcome expectations in realistic terms
f. Confirm verbally or in writing his consent for the operative procedure

Individualized patient care problems call for more specific outcome criteria. For example, a patient experiencing preoperative anxiety and exhibiting physiologic symptoms, including rapid, shallow breathing at a rate of 36 and a rapid pulse rate of 86, might have the following outcome criteria.

- Breathing slowed to + 5 respirations/ minute, compared to patient's normal respiration rate (as charted preoperatively on vital sign graph)
- Pulse slowed to + 10 beats/minute, compared to the patient's normal pulse rate

It is essential for these outcome criteria to be specifically identified for each patient in order to evaluate the effects of individualized nursing care.

◆ Collection of data

Data are collected during or after nursing interventions have been carried out. If outcome criteria have been individualized and written in measurable terms, data collection is greatly facilitated.

In the previous example regarding symptoms of preoperative anxiety, the nurse would measure the patient's pulse (P) and respiration rate (R). In fact, any member of the health care team could collect this data and the measurement would be consistent.

◆ Comparison of data to outcome criteria

Collected data are compared to outcome criteria to determine if expected patient outcomes have been achieved. In this step, the nurse judges whether the nursing interventions were appropriate and attained the desired outcomes, or whether further planning and interventions will be necessary.

In the previous example, if the patient's normal vital signs included a P = 70-72/min and R = 20-22/min, and measurement of vital signs following the nursing intervention were P = 77 and R = 26, the nurse could conclude that the interventions were appropriate and effective. If the data collected did not support the expected outcomes, the nurse would reassess the interventions and determine the need for further action, if any.

◆ Communication of findings

Communication of the status of outcome achievement is essential in providing for continuity of care. Such communication includes:

- Verbally informing other health care team members concerning the findings.
- Discussing patient outcomes and recommending further interventions, if appropriate.
- Documenting patient responses to nursing interventions. (Such documentation affirms that the final step of the nursing process has been completed.)

INTRAOPERATIVE NURSING ACTIVITIES

Intraoperatively, the same steps of the nursing care evaluation process described above are followed. Often, however, the expected outcome criteria for the intraoperative phase are identified during the initial preoperative planning stage.

The intraoperative evaluation process includes the following considerations.

◆ Development of outcome criteria

Outcome criteria established for evaluating intraoperative nursing interventions also should be individualized to the patient. Such individualized criteria would be illustrated in the case of a 51-year-old female who is being placed in the prone position for a multiple bone marrow aspiration. An outcome for this patient and the related outcome criteria might include, but would not be limited to:

- Expected Outcome: Patient is free from injury related to positioning.
- Outcome Criteria:
  a. Pedal and radial pulses are the same rate and quality before and after positioning.
  b. Vital signs 10 minutes after positioning are within + 10% of the measurements taken prior to positioning.

◆ Collection of data

Collection of data regarding the above example would include:

- Palpation and measurement of pulses by the nurse immediately after positioning
- Measurement of all vital signs by the anesthesia care provider 10 minutes after positioning has been completed

◆ Comparison of data to outcome criteria

In the above example, comparison of pre- and post-positioning pedal pulses and vital signs would reveal whether nursing interventions related to safe positioning were appropriate and effective.

If the outcome criteria were not met, it might not be because the nursing interventions were inappropriate. For example, in Criterion "b" listed above, other factors could result in an indication of unstable vital signs 10 minutes after positioning. However, failure to achieve the expected outcome should alert the nurse to recheck positioning.

◆ Communication of findings

Communication of the evaluation findings would include:

- Verbally alerting team members to the findings
- Documenting on the intraoperative record the pulse rates and vital signs measured immediately prior to positioning and after positioning

POSTOPERATIVE NURSING ACTIVITIES

Postoperatively, the nurse evaluates those expected outcomes related to the care that is given during this final phase, in addition to the care provided throughout the surgical procedure. The postoperative evaluation process includes the following considerations.

◆ Time frame in which the patient outcome is to be achieved

Often, the specific criterion for measuring outcomes requires the patient to be responsive; therefore, the time frame for evaluation is frequently established during for the postoperative period. An example of such a time frame is included below.

- Expected Outcome: Patient is free from neuromuscular complications 24 hours postoperatively.
- Outcome Criteria:
  a. Range of motion of extremities equal to range of motion measured preoperatively
  b. Absence of numbness
  c. Absence of joint pain

◆ Collection of data

In the above example, data collection would include such activities as:

- Physical assessment of the patient
- Interview with the patient
- Review of the chart regarding the patient's health status prior to the surgical intervention

◆ Comparison of data collected to observed patient outcomes

In the above example, this comparison would be achieved by analyzing the actual neuromuscular functioning of the patient in the immediate 24-hour postoperative period and then comparing this data with the neuromuscular function the patient possessed at the time of the preoperative assessment.

◆ Communication regarding the status of outcome attainment

As in the other two phases, communication provides the link in the continuity of care. In the previous example, additional nursing actions that may be necessary, if the expected outcome criteria are not met, will become the responsibility of the postanesthesia nursing staff and/or the staff on the inpatient unit. However, the perioperative nurse also may benefit from the outcome findings by adjusting interventions for future patients. In this way, measuring nursing care outcomes becomes an important link in the overall quality improvement process.

EVALUATING THE QUALITY OF NURSING CARE

In measuring quality of nursing care or overall effectiveness of care, it is important not only to measure the current level of care provided, but also to focus on whether continuous improvement in care and services are being achieved. Methods of examining the level of effectiveness may include review and evaluation of care, monitoring or measuring patterns/trends, peer review, performance evaluation, customer satisfaction surveys/focus groups, and conducting research studies to validate effectiveness of care and/or services. In some organizations, case managers and/or outcome management personnel review patient outcomes in collaboration with other members of the health care team to improve consistency and continuity of care and to measure success of patient outcomes. Critical pathways may be used to define patient outcomes that can be expected at each point in the patient's continuum of care and then used as a measurement by which to compare actual outcomes achieved.

The Joint Commission on Accreditation of Healthcare Organizations (JCAHO) includes in its review process measuring effectiveness through performance focused standards. JCAHO defines the characteristics of quality performance as "Doing the Right Thing," which includes efficacy and appropriateness of care and "Doing the Right Thing Well." This includes the availability of appropriate care, the timeliness of the delivery, and the effectiveness and continuity of care. The care is to be delivered safely, efficiently, and in a respectful and caring manner. This definition indicates the need to go beyond measuring the effectiveness of quality care provided to individual patients. All systems and processes that support or affect the care given must be examined using the above definitions as guidelines.

Because systems and processes rarely involve one unit, department, or group of people, it is necessary for members of different units, departments, or disciplines to collaborate in measuring and redesigning, as necessary, the systems and services that will ultimately provide the level of quality care and service expected. These groups are frequently called cross-functional or multidisciplinary teams.

Any problem-solving process can be used to measure performance indicators. Several models are available, such as the Ten Step Model and the Plan-Do-Check-Act Cycle. Another possible process for examining effectiveness has the following eight steps.

- Identify the expected outcome (goal or improvement to be made).
- Establish outcome criteria that will serve as indicators that the standard has been achieved.
- Collect and prioritize data (actual measuring of the important criteria or aspects of care).
- Compare findings of measurement to outcome standards and criteria.
- Design and implement action plans aimed at improving care or services and resolving problems.
- Reinstitute steps 3 and 4 above as appropriate.
- Identify any further action/follow-up needed.
- Document and communicate findings.

Through participation in the process described above, the perioperative nurse accepts accountability for continuous improvement of the care and services provided to perioperative patients.

SUMMARY

The quality of nursing care is a continuum that ranges from inadequate to excellent. A hospital's quality improvement program is established to ensure that the care provided is the best possible for each individual patient. This is accomplished by objectively and systematically assessing and evaluating the quality and appropriateness of patient care and by seeking methods to continuously improve care and to resolve any problems in the overall perioperative process that may be identified.

CASE STUDIES

Case Study: Mr. V

Mr. V, who is 73 years old, is scheduled for removal of a left cataract as an outpatient in the ambulatory surgery unit. Mr. V lives with his wife, age 69. The patient arrives in the preoperative assessment area accompanied only by the taxi driver who has brought him to the ambulatory surgery unit.

Mr. V speaks only Spanish. The taxi driver explains that the patient did not want to come to the hospital for surgery; he only went to the doctor's office to get a pair of glasses so that he could see better. However, Mr. V's wife "talked him into coming so his eyes would get better." The taxi driver does not know the V family. He was dispatched to their home because he speaks Spanish. The taxi company is planning to dispatch this driver again to take Mr. V home after he has had surgery.

The nurses in the preoperative assessment area are concerned about Mr. V's knowledge of his surgical procedure, as well as the lack of arrangements for his transportation home with an individual who is willing to take responsibility for his care during the trip. Based on these concerns, the nurses have identified the following patient care outcomes.

- *Outcome 1:* Patient is able to communicate with

health care team members throughout the perioperative period.

- *Outcome 2:* Patient verbalizes knowledge of the physiological response to surgical intervention.
- *Outcome 3:* Patient is safely transported home postoperatively.

Ms. A, RN, one of the PACU nurses in ambulatory care, serves as an interpreter during the perioperative phases. Mr. V has talked freely with Ms. A about his surgery. She has been able to ascertain that the patient understands what the surgical procedure involves and why the doctor has stated that the surgery is necessary. Mr. V also has indicated that his wife has arthritis and did not come to the hospital with him because it is "too hard for her to get around."

The patient states that his 32-year-old daughter, who lives with her parents, will return home from work that afternoon. However, after a lengthy discussion with Ms. A, Mr. V still does not indicate an understanding of the fact that he will need help when he arrives home, because he will have one eye bandaged and may not be able to get around the house as easily as before.

Points to Consider

- What outcome criteria would be appropriate for evaluating:
  a. Patient care Outcome 1?
  b. Patient care Outcome 2?
  c. Patient care Outcome 3?
- What additional data might be helpful in determining if Outcome 1 has been achieved?
- Compare the data provided to determine if Outcome 2 has been met.
- What nursing actions would be necessary upon reassessment of Outcome 2?
- Identify methods of collecting data that would be related to Outcome 3.

Discussion of Points to Consider

Your responses should have included the following points:

- Outcome criteria for the three identified patient outcomes:

  Outcome 1: Patient is able to communicate with health care team members throughout the perioperative period.

  Outcome Criteria:
  - Patient will communicate through an interpreter.
  - Patient will ask questions about surgery and perioperative care.
  - Patient will respond appropriately to directions given during the perioperative experience.
  - Patient will verbalize understanding of postoperative instructions.

  Outcome 2: Patient verbalizes knowledge of the physiological response to the surgical intervention.

  Outcome Criteria:
  - Patient will describe his understanding of the surgical procedure in his own words.
  - Patient will verbalize his understanding of restrictions in postoperative period related to the surgery.
  - Patient will discuss his concerns related to the surgical procedure.
  - Patient will verbalize expectations for the outcome of cataract surgery.

  Outcome 3: Patient is safely transported home postoperatively.

  Outcome Criteria:
  - Patient will be escorted home by individual(s) who will assume responsibility for his care, such as a family member, friend, or a person with medical background.
  - Patient will arrive home with eye dressing intact.
  - Patient will arrive home without accidents or physical injury.

Additional data that might be helpful in determining if Outcome 1 has been achieved:

- Patient's description of surgical procedure
- Description of the patient's behavioral responses to directions given to him
- Patient's specific responses to questions regarding his understanding of postoperative instructions

Comparison of the data provided to determine if Outcome 2 has been met:

- Based on the data provided in the case study, the expected outcomes have only partially been achieved. According to Ms. A, Mr. V is able to describe his surgery but is unable to verify that he understands the need for assistance because of impaired vision. In addition, other postoperative restrictions have not been mentioned. The data do not indicate that the remaining outcome criteria have been met.

Nursing actions that would be necessary upon reassessment of Outcome 2:

- Have patient verify signature.
- Document verification in perioperative record.
- Question patient through an interpreter regarding his concerns and allow time for discussion/teaching.
- Question patient through an interpreter regarding his expectations related to the surgical outcome.
- Document interventions and patient responses.
- Contact patient's surgeon if necessary to increase patient's knowledge and level of understanding.

Methods of collecting data that would be related to Outcome 3:

- Identification of person escorting patient home.
- Postoperative follow-up telephone call to patient's home.
- Family member's description of eye dressings.
- Patient's verbal response to questions regarding trip home and his physiological/psychological state.

Case Study: Mrs. M

Mrs. M, a 32-year-old housewife, has undergone a total pelvic exenteration, with vaginal reconstruction using myocutaneous flaps from the inner portion of both thighs. The patient was on the OR bed for 9 hours and 20 minutes.

The nurses who are planning Mrs. M's perioperative care list several essential patient care outcomes. Among these outcomes are the following:

- *Outcome 1*: The patient is free from injury related to positioning.
- *Outcome 2:* The patient is free from injury related to electrical hazards.
- *Outcome 3:* The patient's skin integrity is maintained.

Before positioning for the operative procedure, a thermal pad was placed on the mattress, covered by an "egg-crate" pad. One layer of a muslin sheet was placed over the padding. Mrs. M was placed on the OR bed so that her buttocks aligned with the break of the bed. A 1-inch thick foam pad also was placed under the sacrum to provide additional padding, as well as to allow for a slight elevation of the rectal area.

After being anesthetized, the patient was placed in a modified lithotomy position using exenteration stirrups, which cradle the lower legs by allowing the entire length of the calves to be supported from 3 inches above the popliteal space down to and including the foot plates that support the feet. These stirrups allow for minimal flexion of the thighs and 25 to 30 degrees abduction of the legs. The entire length of the stirrups were padded with "egg-crate" foam rubber padding. Heel protectors made from the same material were applied to both feet before placing them in the stirrups.

In addition, both arms were abducted to approximately 80 degrees and secured on armboards padded with foam padding. Before and immediately after positioning, strong and regular bilateral radial and pedal pulses were recorded for both feet, at a rate of 68-70 beats/min.

The surgical prep involved a large surface area: the anterior chest and abdomen from bedside to bedside, both groins, mons pubis, perineal area, vagina, and both thighs circumferentially. Because of the extent of the prep, the dispersive ground pad for the electrosurgical generator was placed under the left gluteal area.

Postoperatively, the patient's pedal pulses were strong and regular and registered 70 beats/min. Radial pulses were also strong and regular and registered 66-68 beats/min. Inspection of the patient's skin revealed a reddened area (approximately 5 cm in diameter) located slightly to the left of the coccygeal area. No other reddened areas of the skin were noted. This reddened area was documented on the perioperative record and communicated to the PACU nurse for follow-up observation. Two hours later, the PACU nurse reports that this area is dark red, with blistering over the skin surface.

Points to Consider

- What outcome criteria would be appropriate for:
  - a. Patient care Outcome 1?
  - b. Patient care Outcome 2?
  - c. Patient care Outcome 3?
- What methods would be used to collect data for the identified criteria?
- What changes in physiological status related to the surgical procedure would limit the nurse's ability to collect data for postoperative evaluation of the outcome criteria?
- What data is missing that would be necessary for comparison of these criteria to actual outcomes?
- What further nursing actions would be necessary, based on the degree of achievement of Outcome 3?
- Discuss necessary communication related to the achievement of Outcome 3.

Discussion of Points to Consider

Your responses should have included the following points:

- Outcome criteria for the three identified patient care outcomes:
  Outcome 1: Patient is free from injury related to positioning.
    Outcome Criteria: Physical examination of the patient will demonstrate:
    - No numbness or tingling sensation in limbs during 24-hour postoperative period.
    - Flexion, extension, and rotation of both ankles in 24-hour postoperative period equal to that measured during preoperative assessment.
    - Full range of motion of both arms postoperatively, in accordance with preoperative assessment.
    - Adequate perfusion of extremities, as revealed by: strong and regular pedal pulses, with a rate of 58-80 immediately after positioning and after transfer to PACU bed; and warm to touch, with even coloration and absence of redness.

  Outcome 2: Patient is free from injury related to electrical hazards.
    Outcome Criteria:
    - No reddened skin areas are noted under dispersive electrode or ECG electrodes.
    - No swelling is noted under dispersive electrode or ECG electrodes.

  Outcome 3: Patient's skin integrity is maintained.
    Outcome Criterion:
    - The patient will have no evidence of reddened areas 24 hours postoperatively and no breaks in the skin.

Methods of data collection for outcome criteria:

- Observation of range of motion
- Interview of patient related to sensation in extremities
- Palpation of pulses
- Inspection of skin
- Follow-up communication with PACU staff

Limitations in data collection due to physiological changes resulting from surgery:

- The patient's inability to move her legs postoperatively because of the restrictions imposed by the rotated myocutaneous flaps from the inner thighs would limit the nurse's ability to determine if there is impaired mobility/range of motion related to positioning.

Missing data that would be necessary for comparison of criteria to outcomes:

- Preoperative status of patient's skin.
- Preoperative range of motion of extremities.

Further nursing actions that would be necessary, due to lack of achievement of Outcomes 3:

- Reporting occurrence to surgeon and other appropriate individuals (ie, risk manager, patient outcomes manager).
- Documentation of appearance of developing a skin breakdown.
- Establishment of new outcome criteria for evaluating patient response to nursing management of skin breakdown.
- Planning and implementation of care related to restoration of skin integrity in coccygeal area.
- Continued monitoring and documentation of healing process.
- Monitoring of placement of electrosurgical dispersive pads in future high-risk patients.

Communication related to the achievement of Outcome 3:

- Documentation on the perioperative record of the reddened area noted postoperatively.
- Verbal communication between OR and PACU staff related to postoperative findings.
- Documentation of the new plan of care.
- Documentation of progress of healing in the patient's medical record.
- Patient care conference to review outcomes of care for Mrs. M and to identify future steps in order to avoid a repeat of this incident.

Case Study: Hospital X OR Turnover Time

Hospital X is a 200-bed hospital with six inpatient operating rooms located in the main hospital building and four outpatient operating rooms located in the professional building adjacent to the hospital. The two buildings are connected with a crosswalk. A wide variety of specialty services are represented by the procedures done in both OR settings, including procedures using the latest technology such as video-assisted laparoscopic procedures. Equipment is shared between the inpatient and outpatient operating rooms. The inpatient OR is staffed for elective procedures Monday through Friday from 7:30 AM to 3:00 PM with two of the operating rooms staffed until 5:30 PM to accommodate elective procedures that start before 2:00 PM but run past 3:00 PM. "On call" staff coverage is provided for urgent/emergent procedures after 5:30 PM on weekdays and on weekends.

Excessive turnover times are identified as contributing to an inefficient OR schedule, underutilized facilities, and dissatisfaction between staff and physicians. A task force representing nursing, anesthesia, surgeons, and administration met to address the issues of turnover time.

The standard definition of turnover time at Hospital X is identified as the time between the point that one patient leaves the operating room to be transported to PACU and the time the next patient enters the operating room to be transferred to the OR bed. Using this definition, turnover time in the inpatient (ie, main) OR was consistently measured to be in excess of 45 minutes with many cases averaging 50 to 90 minutes. Average case length in the main OR is about 1.5 to 2 hours, and an average of 16 to 18 cases are done each day during the elective hours.

The inpatient operating rooms use a case cart system in which central processing provides basic supplies/equipment. Specialty supplies/equipment are added to the case cart by the OR staff before the cart is taken into the OR.

The staffing ratio for most procedures has been 2:1 (that is, one circulating nurse and one scrub nurse for each procedure regardless of patient acuity or complexity of procedure). Occasionally, there has been one extra nurse in addition to the supervisor "floating" between the operating rooms.

Staff responsibilities are as follows:

- The scrub nurse assists with the clean-up procedure, procures and opens supplies, moves in the necessary equipment, scrubs, and begins to set up the instrumentation.
- The circulating nurse and anesthesia personnel transfer the patient to PACU, complete necessary perioperative documentation and charge documents, and assess the next patient.
- Additional assistive personnel consist of the two nursing aides who transport patients, carry specimens to the lab, and clean operating rooms between cases.

Frequently, there are delays related to:

- Delay between the completion of the assessment and transfer of the patient to the OR because the circulating nurse must return to the OR to assist the scrub nurse in completing the case preparation.
- Delays during the intraoperative preparation phase after the patient is brought into the room because of equipment (eg, positioning devices) that has not been collected.
- Delays due to additional circulating duties related to the increased technology used on many of the cases.

Excessive turnover time has increased the length of the surgery schedule, resulting in a decrease in the number of surgeries that are posted during the 7:30 AM to 3:00 PM hours. There also has been an increase in overtime among nursing and anesthesia personnel related to elective procedures running past 5:30 PM.

Dissatisfaction was high among the surgeons related to increased waiting time between cases and increasing difficulty in posting procedures. Frustration of the nursing and anesthesia personnel was high because of the increased overtime and mounting pressure to improve turnover time. It seemed that no matter how "fast or hard" they worked, the turnover time did not change appreciably, while the number of undesired occurrences and mistakes made because of their hurry did increase.

The task force appointed to address the turnover issue identified the following initial continuous quality improvement (CQI) goals:

- *Goal 1:* Turnover time will decrease.
- *Goal 2:* Available posting time will increase.
- *Goal 3:* Physician, nursing, and anesthesia dissatisfaction related to problems associated with excessive turnover time will decrease.

Points to Consider

- What additional goals might have been identified by the task force?
- What outcome criteria would be appropriate for evaluating?
  a. Goal 1?
  b. Goal 2?
  c. Goal 3?
- What additional data collection methods other than general details/description of the current system in place and the subsequent problems might be helpful in deciding how to address the three goals set by the task force, as well as how to actually measure progress toward meeting those goals?
- Identify potential action steps that the task force might implement in their plan to correct the problem of excessive turnover time.
- What communication regarding findings of the task force would be appropriate?

Discussion of Points to Consider

Your responses should have included the following points:

- Additional goals that might have been identified by the task force are:
  - Overtime of anesthesia and nursing staff will decrease.
  - Number of undesired occurrences/mistakes will decrease.
- Outcome criteria for the three identified CQI goals:
  Goal 1: Turnover time will decrease.
  Outcome Criterion: Turnover time will average 10 to 20 minutes between cases.
  Goal 2: Available posting time will increase.
  Outcome Criterion: Available elective schedule time will accommodate an average of 22 to 26 cases to be posted daily.
  Goal 3: Physician, nursing, and anesthesia dissatisfaction related to problems associated with excessive turnover time will decrease.
  Outcome Criteria:
  - Physicians will verbalize satisfaction regarding a decrease in waiting time between cases and increased ability to post elective procedures between 7:30 AM and 5:30 PM.
  - Nursing staff members will verbalize satisfaction related to decreased overtime and decreased number of undesired occurrences/mistakes made.
  - Anesthesia staff members will verbalize satisfaction related to decreased overtime and decreased number of undesired occurrences/mistakes made.

Additional data collection methods that could be helpful in deciding how to address the three goals set by the task force as well as how to actually measure progress toward meeting those goals could include:

- Measurement of dissatisfaction levels of physicians, nursing staff, and anesthesia staff before and after implementation of the action plan to address turnover time.
- Measurement of the amount of overtime accrued by nursing and anesthesia staff before and after implementation of the action plan.
- Measurement of the number of undesired occurrences/mistakes reported before and after implementation of the plan.
- Research of community practice/standards and literature related to standards for turnover time, methods used to decrease turnover, and acuity systems in place to assist in staffing decisions.

Potential action steps that the task force might recommend in their plan to correct the problems of excessive turnover time could include:

- Identify equipment necessary to eliminate the need to transport frequently used items back and forth between day surgery and the main OR.
- Requesting an allocation of funds to purchase necessary equipment, justifying request through a cost-benefit analysis (ie, loss of 4 to 8 cases/day because of turnover time versus cost of equipment).
- Recommending cross training of assistive personnel to include preparing case carts with necessary supplies/equipment between cases.
- Evaluating the need for additional assistive personnel to help with preparation of case carts, transport of patients and specimens, and cleaning of operating rooms.
- Implementing an acuity system to assist in determining adequate staffing needed.
- Evaluating need for additional nursing staff based on comparison of current staffing to staffing recommended by the acuity system chosen.
- Implementing an evaluation plan that will measure goal achievement at time intervals of 1 month, 3 months, and 6 months to determine what changes in the action plan or additional measures need to be taken based on findings.

Appropriate communication regarding findings of the task force include:

- Reporting to physicians, nursing, and anesthesia staff findings of the task force as well as action steps recommended to solve turnover dilemma.
- Posting turnover times weekly to allow everyone to monitor progress related to an action plan.
- Submitting written description of a problem and action plan throughout the appropriate channels as identified in the hospital CQI plan.

SUGGESTED LEARNING ACTIVITIES

If you are unsure of your level of expertise in regard to evaluating the effectiveness of the plan of care, using some or all of the following learning activities will be helpful in your self-assessment process.

- ◆ Spend time in the PACU or on one of the nursing units, reviewing assessment data and identified patient outcome standards that are documented in the charts of patients with complex health problems. Practice writing what you think would be appropriate outcome criteria for each of the identified standards. Discuss the outcome criteria that you have written with a colleague.

- Have a colleague or your supervisor critique the evaluation activities (eg, written outcome criteria, documented outcomes, adjustments in the plan of care) that you perform in caring for the patients to whom you are assigned.
- Review the evaluation activities of your colleagues for ideas and examples of different evaluation approaches.
- Form a discussion group with other colleagues in order to identify high-risk/high-incident surgical procedures in your OR. Develop an extensive list of outcome criteria for each of AORN's "Patient Outcomes: Standards for Perioperative Care" as they relate to the high-risk/high-incident surgical procedures you have identified.
- Volunteer to serve on a task force or focus group to address quality improvements that need to be made. Volunteer to help write the goals and outcome criteria by which the group will evaluate achievements.
- Participate in the data collection and evaluation process of the task force to practice your skills at comparing written criteria to the actual outcomes achieved.

RECOMMENDED STUDY MATERIALS

AORN, *Standards, Recommended Practices, and Guidelines* (Denver: AORN, Inc, 2002).

Ireson, C L, "Critical Pathways: Effectiveness in Achieving Patient Outcomes," *Journal of Nursing Administration* 27 (June 1997) 16-23.

JCAHO, *2002 Comprehensive Accreditation Manual for Hospitals* (Oakbrook Terrace, Ill: Joint Commission on Accreditation of Healthcare Organizations, 2002).

Killen A R, "The prevalence of perioperative nurse clinical judgments," *AORN Journal* 65 (1) (January 1997) 101-108.

Kneedler, J A; G H Dodge, eds, *Perioperative Patient Care: The Nursing Perspective,* third ed (Boston: Jones and Bartlett, 1994).

Lbarra, V, "Clinical pathways in the perioperative setting," *Nursing Case Management* 2 (3) (May/June 1997) 97-106.

May, CA; Schraeder, C; Britt, T, *Managed Care and Case Management: Roles for Professional Nursing* (Washington, DC: American Nurses Publishing, 1996).

Wammack, I, et al, "Outcomes assessment of total hip and total knee arthroplasty: Critical pathways, variance analysis, and continuous quality improvement," *Clinical Nurse Specialist* 12 (3) (May 1998) 122-131.

CHAPTER 11: ORGANIZE AND COORDINATE TEAM MEMBERS, SUPPLIES, EQUIPMENT, AND SUPPORT SERVICES

Mary Lynne Weemering, RN, MSN, CNOR

Nursing assessment in the perioperative setting is data gathering about the patient in order to individualize care with the ultimate objective of a positive patient outcome. Because it is the responsibility of the perioperative nurse to organize and coordinate team members, supplies, equipment, and support services, data about the patient must not only be gathered, but also must be analyzed and integrated into an overall plan. A well-organized plan contributes to a safe environment for the patient and provides the optimum setting for a positive outcome. Factors that affect the organizing process include the availability of supplies, equipment, and instruments and also include the preferences of the physician. The perioperative nurse must give consideration to fiscal management of both supplies and human resources. The need for cost-effectiveness must be balanced with safe patient care.

The patient, family, and/or significant other are important sources of information during data gathering, and their involvement may help to establish a trusting relationship between the patient and the nurse. The amount of involvement depends on the patient's condition and the unique circumstances surrounding each patient. Although teaching may be appropriate in other settings, it must be used with caution in the assessment period due to the potential for high anxiety of the patient. Information sharing is more likely to be successful and appropriate for the patient/family and also will enable informed decision making. There are circumstances when the patient chooses to decline surgical intervention at this stage, and it is incumbent that the perioperative nurse support the patient's decision and be an advocate.

In addition to information gathered from the patient, family, and/or significant other, the perioperative nurse must review the medical record for a comprehensive view. The medical record should contain a history/physical and diagnostic studies that provide insight into the patient's overall condition. After all pertinent information is gathered and analyzed, it must be shared to be the most useful. Information sharing in the form of collaboration, communication, and coordination is necessary for continuity of care to occur. This process of information sharing must be critically performed so that appropriate information can be shared with team members.

LEARNING OBJECTIVES

This chapter pertains to the organization and coordination of team members, supplies, equipment, and support services necessary for perioperative patient care. The step-by-step activities are listed in such a way as to help the perioperative nurse gain organizational skills. This chapter does not focus on the administrative and/or the managerial functions that occur in the OR.

Upon completion of this chapter, the perioperative nurse should be able to:

1. Analyze and integrate assessment findings into a plan of care.

2. Provide a safe environment that contributes to a positive patient outcome.

3. Organize and coordinate team members and equipment to meet the unique needs of the patient.

4. Collaborate with health care team members to ensure continuity of care.

TASK STATEMENT; AREAS OF KNOWLEDGE AND SKILL

Task Statement

Organize and coordinate team members, supplies, equipment, and support services to maintain an efficient, effective, and safe environment, accomplished by teaching, directing, delegating, communicating, and collaborating with health care team members.

Areas of Knowledge

K-4 Pharmacology and anesthetic agents
K-5 Pain management
K-6 Principles of wound healing
K-8 Preoperative patient preparation activities
K-9 Surgical, anesthetic, and other perioperative interventions
K-12 Principles of positioning
K-13 Ergonomics and body mechanics
K-14 Transfer and transport techniques and equipment
K-15 Risks for injury, including but not limited to, skin, positioning, and retained foreign body
K-16 Emergency procedures (eg, CPR, MH)
K-17 Postoperative complications
K-18 Defining characteristics of impending patient physiologic crisis
K-29 Emergency operative procedures
K-20 Sociology (eg, cultural and ethnic influences, family patterns, spirituality and related practices)
K-21 Communication theories and techniques
K-22 Behavioral responses to the surgical experience
K-24 Theories of and resources for patient/family education
K-25 *Perioperative Nursing Data Set* (PNDS)
K-26 Requirements for handling of specimens
K-27 Microbiology and infection control
K-28 Standard and transmission-based precautions
K-29 Potential hazards in the perioperative environment
K-30 Interventions to optimize safety
K-31 Technologies and equipment relating to perioperative practice
K-32 Environmental parameters (eg, temperature, humidity, air exchange)
K-33 Principles of sterilization and disinfection
K-34 Protective barrier materials
K-37 Principles of product evaluation, cost-containment, and resource management
K-35 Packaging materials
K-36 Principles of equipment inspection, maintenance, and repair
K-38 Emergency preparedness (eg, fire, disaster)
K-39 Patient rights and responsibilities
K-40 Legal responsibilities and implications for patient care
K-42 Nursing research and evidence-based practice
K-43 "ANA Code of Ethics for Nurses with Explications for Perioperative Nurses"
K-44 Regulatory standards and voluntary guidelines
K-45 AORN *Standards, Recommended Practices, and Guidelines*
K-46 AORN position statements (eg, bloodborne pathogens, do-not-resuscitate orders [DNR])
K-47 Principles of problem solving
K-48 Quality improvement principles
K-50 Defining characteristics of impaired individuals (eg, substance abuse, psychological disturbance, compromised performance)
K-51 Inappropriate workplace behaviors (eg, harassment, workplace violence)
K-52 Defining characteristics of domestic abuse (eg, child, elder, partner/spouse)
K-53 Rules, responsibilities, and duties of health care team members and internal and external support service personnel
K-54 Organ procurement
K-55 Credentialing standards and clinical privileges
K-56 Implants (eg, handling, tracking, sterilization)
K-57 Health care trends and issues

Areas of Skill

S-1 Confirming patient identity, operative site, and procedure
S-2 Collecting, analyzing, and prioritizing patient data
S-3 Using health assessment techniques (eg, interview, observation, auscultation, palpation, percussion)
S-4 Communicating effectively (verbal and nonverbal)
S-5 Advocating and protecting patient rights
S-6 Evaluating environment for discharge care
S-7 Assessing and managing pain
S-8 Assessing for potential abuse (eg, substance, domestic)
S-9 Assessing readiness to learn, knowledge level, and preferred learning style
S-10 Identifying barriers to learning
S-12 Identifying cultural, spiritual, and ethnic issues in care
S-13 Identifying age-specific needs
S-15 Collaborating with other members on the health care team
S-16 Applying AORN *Standards, Recommended Practices, and Guidelines*

S-17 Applying the *Perioperative Nursing Data Set* (PNDS)
S-18 Delineating and communicating measurable patient outcomes
S-19 Participating in quality improvement activities
S-20 Maintaining accurate patient records
S-21 Protecting patients and members of the health care team from hazardous conditions
S-22 Providing evidence-based care
S-23 Applying regulatory standards and voluntary guidelines
S-25 Apply principles of and participate in cost containment, product evaluation, and resource management
S-26 Incorporating community and institutional resources into plan of care
S-27 Delegating interventions and/or assigning tasks
S-28 Adapting to changing situations and technologies
S-29 Performing nursing interventions
S-32 Applying principles and techniques of transport, transfer, and positioning
S-33 Anticipating the needs for equipment, supplies, and personnel
S-34 Applying principles and techniques of body mechanics/ergonomics
S-35 Maintaining the dignity, modesty, and privacy of the patient and protecting the confidentiality of patient information
S-37 Applying principles of sterilization and disinfection
S-38 Applying principles of environmental cleaning
S-39 Maintaining a sterile field
S-40 Preparing the surgical site
S-43 Controlling environmental noise
S-44 Testing and using equipment
S-45 Monitoring physiological parameters
S-46 Anticipating and evaluating the effects of pharmacological and anesthetic agents
S-47 Documenting maintenance of a safe environment
S-48 Detecting significant changes in the environment
S-49 Preparing and handling specimens for diagnostic evaluation
S-50 Adapting to special and unusual needs
S-51 Identifying and communicating changes in patient status
S-53 Educating, mentoring, and supervising health care team members
S-54 Recognizing impaired behavior in patients, family, and staff members and responding appropriately
S-55 Recognizing personal limitations and seeking assistance as needed
S-57 Performing sterilization procedures and conducting monitoring techniques (eg, chemical, biological monitoring, and mechanical indicators)
S-58 Identifying appropriate packaging materials for sterilization
S-60 Directing health care team members in emergency situations
S-62 Setting priorities
S-63 Evaluating self and others according to goals and standards
S-65 Applying ethical principles
S-68 Performing required counts
S-69 Recording devices implanted or explanted during procedures
S-70 Classifying the surgical wound
S-71 Securing patient belongings and valuables

PREOPERATIVE NURSING ACTIVITIES

The preoperative phase of the surgical experience begins with the decision for surgery and ends when the patient is transferred into the OR. The organization and coordination of human and material resources includes, but is not limited to, the activities listed below. Keep in mind that these activities are not all inclusive because there are administrative and managerial nursing considerations that are not discussed in this chapter (eg, fiscal accountability, staffing requirements, quality management, policy development, personnel management, group process, competency issues, risk management, staff development). The following are activities that a perioperative nurse would generally do in the course of a surgical procedure.

- Ensure that appropriate instruments, equipment, accessories, and implantable devices are available and functioning properly before they are actually needed.
- Collaborate with the admitting nurses to ensure continuity of care.
- Participate or delegate the task of updating physician preference cards.
- Inform support team members of individual needs of the patient.
- Arrange for interdepartmental services (eg, radiology) if needed.
- Open sterile supplies and equipment based on scheduled surgery.
- Interview the patient/family and provide information as appropriate.

- Act as the patient advocate.
- Review the medical record for completeness.
- Ensure correct patient identification in conjunction with the physician.
- Clarify correct surgical site and side with the patient.
- Collaborate with the anesthesia care provider to review the plan.
- Transport the patient to the correct operating room.

INTRAOPERATIVE NURSING ACTIVITIES

The intraoperative phase begins when the patient is transferred onto the operating bed and ends when the patient is transported to postanesthesia recovery area.

- Transfer the patient to the OR bed.
- Assist with anesthesia induction.
- Verify correct site/side again before the incision is made.
- Position patient based on identified surgery.
- Insert indwelling catheter as needed.
- Assist anesthesia care provider to insert any central lines, as needed.
- Count instruments, sharps, and sponges with the scrubbed person before the incision is made.
- Apply a tourniquet(s) as indicated.
- Apply sequential compression device as indicated.
- Apply electrosurgical return electrode (ie, grounding pad) as indicated.
- Apply forced air blanket to prevent hypothermia, as indicated.
- Prepare the identified surgical site with appropriate hair removal as indicated and apply skin antiseptic.
- Connect appropriate equipment/accessories for the scrubbed team.
- Practice standard and transmission-based precautions continuously.
- Provide any medications, blood/blood products, additional instruments, implantable devices, or other items as needed during the surgery.
- Communicate with the family.
- Ensure bed space for postanesthesia recovery.
- Document nursing activities and any other required information including any adverse events.
- Receive tissue specimens from the scrubbed team, and ensure the specimen is transported to the appropriate department for examination.
- Count instruments/sharps/sponges to ensure that all are received back from the sterile field.
- Apply dressings or assist with cast application as indicated.
- Remove any items that are no longer needed from the patient at the conclusion of the surgery (eg, the return electrode for electrosurgery).
- Inspect the patient's skin for intactness.
- Transfer patient to a gurney or bed as indicated.
- Transport the patient to the identified postanesthesia recovery area.

POSTOPERATIVE NURSING ACTIVITIES

The postoperative phase begins when the patient is admitted to the postanesthesia care unit and ends with the resolution of the surgical sequelae.

- Communicate pertinent patient information to the receiving nurse to ensure continuity of care.
- Delegate and/or participate in OR disinfection using principles of standard precautions.
- Transport (or delegate the task) contaminated instruments to the decontamination area.
- Ready the OR for subsequent procedures.

SUMMARY

The perioperative nurse uses many skills when organizing and coordinating the care of the patient during his or her surgical experience and providing a safe environment for that patient. These skills include assessment; gathering of data; organizing supplies, equipment, and team members; and collaborating with all members of the health care team to ensure continuity of care for the patient.

CASE STUDIES

Case Study: Mr. P

Mr. P is an 89-year-old male who arrived at the hospital by ambulance from an extended care facility where he had fallen and was unable to get up or bear weight on his left leg. Mr. P is a widower and is accompanied by his adult son. He has pain in the left groin and was placed in Buck's traction after radiologic studies showed that he had sustained an intertrochanteric fracture of the left hip. Since hospitalization, Mr. P has become confused. He is scheduled for open reduction internal fixation of the left hip with compression hip system. The hospital does not stock the compression hip system that the orthopedic surgeon desires to use. How would you organize this pending surgery?

Points to Consider

- How do you arrange for the compression hip system?
- The patient is in Buck's traction; how should the patient be transported to the OR?
- A powered drill will be needed; how is the drill powered?
- The patient is confused; who should sign the consent?
- The patient is immobile; how will the patient be moved onto the OR bed?
- A fracture table will be needed; how will it be configured and by whom?
- Fluoroscopy will be used; how is this arranged and what protection should be arranged?
- What kind of anesthesia is likely to be administered?
- The patient likely will be placed directly into his hospital bed; who will prepare the bed?

Discussion of Points to Consider

- If the hospital does not stock a particular fixation system, the manufacturer's representative should be called to arrange for delivery of the system. The system may need to be sterilized; therefore, collaboration with the sterilization department is important.
- The patient is in Buck's traction; therefore, the patient must be transported via bed. You must mobilize enough staff to bring a patient via bed.
- Powered drills use electric, battery, or nitrogen for power. You must consult the physician's preference card to determine which drill he prefers, and then you must find and prepare it.
- When a patient is confused and cannot competently sign the consent, state laws and hospital policy should determine who has authority to consent to the surgery. In this case, the patient was lucid prior to the fall and has become confused after hospitalization.
- The patient cannot move himself from his bed to the OR bed. The physician needs to be present to supervise the transfer. You must mobilize enough staff to safely accomplish the transfer of the patient from his bed to the OR bed.
- Fracture tables are configured differently depending on the type of fracture. You should know how to configure the table as part of your orientation to orthopedic surgery or delegate the task to a support person who knows how.
- Fluoroscopy requires use of the C-arm. You should call the radiology department in advance and arrange for a technician to be present for the surgery. You also should provide lead aprons and thyroid shields for all members of the team.
- You should communicate and collaborate with the anesthesia care provider to determine the plan for anesthesia so that you can have the appropriate materials present. Spinal anesthesia is frequently the anesthetic of choice for this type of surgery. You need to assemble enough staff to support the patient in lateral position so that the anesthesia care provider can administer the spinal.
- The postoperative bed needs to be readied, so you need to delegate this task to support personnel.

Case Study: Mrs. M

Mrs. M is scheduled for an elective pelviscopy and possible right ovarian cystectomy for removal of an ovarian cyst. As Mrs. M reaches the holding area, she asks you to allow her to see a Catholic priest before she goes into surgery. The gynecologist is pressing you to get the surgery started because he is late to his office. How would you organize this minimally invasive surgery, and how would you meet the patient's spiritual needs before she is anesthetized?

Points to Consider

- Pelviscopy is an example of minimally invasive surgery; what kind of instruments and equipment will you choose?
- How will you determine that the video equipment is working properly before the patient is moved into the room?
- Where should the CO_2 tank be placed in relation to the patient?
- What kinds of OR bed attachments will be needed for pelviscopy?
- What should you determine about the CO_2 tank before the procedure starts?
- What physiologic monitoring must be closely watched during CO_2 insufflation?
- What will you do to accommodate the patient's request to see a priest and the physician's request to expedite the surgery?
- The patient will be placed in lithotomy position; what should you know about positioning the patient?
- What thermal event is likely to occur during CO_2 insufflation?

Discussion of Points to Consider

- Instruments for minimally invasive surgery include, but are not limited to, assorted size scopes, trocars, insufflation tubing, light cords, camera, and electrosurgical accessories. Some or all of these instruments may be heat sensitive and may require sterilization other than by steam.
- All electrical equipment should be turned on to test for functionality before the patient is moved into the room. All instruments should be visually examined for adequate insulation for protection of the patient against inadvertent electrosurgical burn.
- The CO_2 tank should be placed higher than the patient's abdomen so that backflow of CO_2 can be avoided. A hydrophobic filter should be used to prevent ferrous particles from being transferred from the CO_2 tank into the patient's abdomen.
- The patient will be placed in lithotomy position, so stirrups will be needed. The legs should be elevated and lowered simultaneously and there should be minimal external rotation of the hips.
- The CO_2 tank should be checked for adequate volume of gas before the surgery starts.
- The patient's end tidal CO_2 should be closely monitored due to the increased risk of hypercarbia.
- The patient's request to see a priest should be honored in spite of the pressure to start the surgery. Perhaps there is a hospital chaplain that could meet the patient's need if a priest is not in the hospital.
- CO_2 insufflation is known to contribute to hypothermia, so it is important that the patient is protected to prevent the event and monitored to watch for trends toward this event.

SUGGESTED LEARNING ACTIVITIES

◆ Review cases you have participated in within the last week and evaluate the care you provided. Are there areas of organization or coordination that you need to improve?

◆ Seek out a peer whose work you respect and ask him or her to evaluate your organizational and coordination skills. Ask this person to identify how he or she plans for a case.

◆ Seek out a surgeon, anesthesia care provider, or nurse colleague whose opinion you respect and ask him or her for an assessment of how cases you have worked with that person on have gone. Are there areas that he or she feels you need to work on?

◆ Work with a mentor who demonstrates strong organizational and coordination skills.

◆ Review recent cases that have not gone well. How could you have anticipated or planned for these cases better. What would you have done differently?

RECOMMENDED STUDY MATERIALS

AORN, *Standards, Recommended Practices, and Guidelines* (Denver: AORN, Inc, 2002).

Fortunato, N H, ed, *Berry & Kohn's Operating Room Technique*, ninth ed (St Louis: Mosby, Inc, 2000).

Meeker, M H; Rothrock, J C, *Alexander's Care of the Patient in Surgery,* 12th ed (St Louis: Mosby, Inc, 2002).

CHAPTER 12: COMMUNICATE PATIENT INFORMATION

Rose Moss, RN, MN, CNOR

Effective communication has always been an integral aspect of the nurse/patient relationship, especially for the surgical patient and his/her family or significant others. Today, the nurse faces an increasingly complex health care system, due to the rapid changes in technology as well as the increasingly culturally diverse patient population. Technological advances in electronics have had a significant impact on the concept of communication, which is accentuated in the health care setting. Not that long ago, patients looked to health care providers as their main source of information. In addition, it was not that many years ago that a registered nurse from the operating room visited hospitalized patients preoperatively to conduct an assessment and provide critical instructions. Today, general health care information is available to the general public from a number of means, such as television, user-friendly interactive web sites, professional organizations, public associations, as well as literature found in many public places. With the focus on economics in health care today, preoperative assessment and instruction, and also postoperative follow-up are conducted via the telephone.

There are two other trends in health care today that affect effective communication. First, there is an increase in the number of multicultural patients being treated in health care facilities today. Therefore, knowledge of cultural diversity issues is critical in all nursing specialties, but especially in the perioperative setting, where cultural differences may exist regarding blood or organ donation, disposal of body parts, and postmortem care, to name only a few. Secondly, the nurse must practice effective communication skills while simultaneously safeguarding the patient's right to privacy. Patients trust nurses to hold all information in confidence, as the right to privacy is an inalienable human right.

All of the trends and considerations noted above reinforce the importance of effective communication skills in the perioperative setting, within today's dynamic health care environment. The professional perioperative nurse must know and practice effective communication skills with patients, family, and significant others to establish and maintain a therapeutic relationship. The professional nurse should have the time needed to meet the patient's need for communication through a health care environment that supports the delegation of technical tasks. There are many benefits of effectual nurse/patient communication, including:

- provision of vital information to assist the patient, family, or significant others in making thoughtful decisions;
- increase in the patient's sense of responsibility and control; and
- promotion of self-care and decision making.

This chapter reviews the core concepts and principles of communication as they relate to professional perioperative nursing practice and improved patient outcomes. Communication is one of the key components in the development of a therapeutic, caring relationship for the surgical patient. In addition, examples of information to be communicated to the patient, family, and significant others related to the nursing activities throughout all phases of the patient's surgical journey, along with the related perioperative nursing competencies, are presented. Case studies are provided to assist the perioperative nurse in applying the principles of effective communication and key nursing considerations.

LEARNING OBJECTIVES

Professional registered nurses preparing for the certification exam in perioperative nursing should include the areas of requisite knowledge and skills to establish and maintain a therapeutic relationship through effective communication. Upon completion of this chapter, the nurse should be able to:

1. Describe the concept of communication.

2. Discuss effective communication skills as an integrated aspect of perioperative nursing practice.

3. State the impact of cultural diversity and confidentiality issues on effective communication.

4. Identify information to be communicated to patients, families, and significant others undergoing surgical intervention or invasive procedures.

TASK STATEMENT; AREAS OF KNOWLEDGE AND SKILL

Task Statement

Communicate patient information to promote continuity of care (eg, family, PACU, ICU, patient unit).

The professional perioperative nurse uses effective communication skills to convey pertinent information to the patient and others (eg, family or significant others and other professionals involved in the care of the patient, such as postanesthesia care unit [PACU], intensive care unit [ICU], and patient care unit staff) to promote continuity of care and positive patient outcomes. In today's dynamic health care environment, including respect for cultural diversities and the patient's right to privacy, effective and appropriate communication takes on even greater significance. Effective communication skills also contribute to the professional growth of the individual nurse and the perioperative specialty. The OR is a unique environment, where such communication is vital for the patient's welfare, and it also can decrease the family's/significant other's stress associated with waiting for a status update in a strange environment.

Areas of Knowledge

- K-1 Health assessment techniques
- K-2 Anatomy and physiology
- K-3 Pathophysiology
- K-4 Pharmacology and anesthetic agents
- K-5 Pain management
- K-6 Principles of wound healing
- K-7 Diagnostic procedures and results
- K-8 Preoperative patient preparation activities
- K-9 Surgical, anesthetic, and other perioperative interventions
- K-10 Expected outcomes related to identified interventions
- K-11 Physiologic responses to the surgical experience
- K-14 Transfer and transport techniques and equipment
- K-15 Risks for injury, including, but not limited to, skin, positioning and retained foreign body
- K-16 Emergency procedures (eg, CPR, MH)
- K-17 Postoperative complications
- K-18 Defining characteristics of impending patient physiologic crisis
- K-19 Emergency operative procedures
- K-20 Sociology (eg, cultural and ethnic influences, family patterns, spirituality and related practices)
- K-21 Communication theories and techniques
- K-22 Behavioral responses to the surgical experience
- K-23 Discharge planning
- K-24 Theories of and resources for patient/family education
- K-25 *Perioperative Nursing Data Set* (PNDS)
- K-27 Microbiology and infection control
- K-28 Standard and transmission-based precautions
- K-29 Potential hazards in the perioperative environment including, but not limited to, chemical, electrical, fire, gas, laser, physical environment, radiologic, extraneous objects
- K-30 Interventions to optimize safety
- K-39 Patient rights and responsibilities
- K-40 Legal responsibilities and implications for patient care
- K-41 Approved nursing diagnoses (eg, NANDA)
- K-43 "ANA Code of Ethics for Nurses with Explications for Perioperative Nurses"
- K-45 AORN *Standards, Recommended Practices, and Guidelines*
- K-46 AORN position statements (eg, bloodborne pathogens, do-not-resuscitate orders [DNR])
- K-47 Principles of problem solving
- K-49 Surgical consent laws and policies
- K-50 Defining characteristics of impaired individuals (eg, substance abuse, psychological disturbance, compromised performance)
- K-52 Defining characteristics of domestic abuse (eg, child, elder, partner/spouse)
- K-54 Organ procurement
- K-55 Credentialing standards and clinical privileges
- K-56 Implants (handling, tracking, sterilization)

Areas of Skill

- S-1 Confirming patient identity, operative site, and procedure
- S-2 Collecting, analyzing, and prioritizing patient data

S-3 Using health assessment techniques (eg, interview, observation, auscultation, palpation, percussion)
S-4 Communicating effectively (verbal and nonverbal)
S-5 Advocating and protecting patient rights
S-6 Evaluating environment for discharge care
S-7 Assessing and managing pain
S-8 Assessing for potential abuse (eg, substance, domestic)
S-9 Assessing readiness to learn, knowledge level, and preferred learning style
S-15 Collaborating with other members on the health care team
S-16 Applying AORN *Standards, Recommended Practices, and Guidelines*
S-17 Applying the *Perioperative Nursing Data Set* (PNDS)
S-18 Delineating and communicating measurable patient outcomes
S-19 Participating in quality improvement activities
S-20 Maintaining accurate patient records
S-22 Providing evidence based care
S-23 Applying regulatory standards and voluntary guidelines
S-27 Delegating interventions and/or assigning tasks
S-28 Adapting to changing situations and technologies
S-30 Documenting all relevant facts and data elements with appropriate terminology
S-31 Recording unusual occurrences and/or variances in care
S-35 Maintaining the dignity, modesty, and privacy of the patient and protecting the confidentiality of patient information
S-46 Anticipating and evaluating the effects of pharmacological and anesthetic agents
S-50 Adapting to special and unusual needs
S-51 Identifying and communicating changes in patient status
S-52 Documenting nursing interventions and patient response
S-53 Educating, mentoring, and supervising health care team members
S-54 Recognizing impaired behavior in patients, family, and staff and responding appropriately
S-56 Measuring, evaluating, and documenting patient outcomes
S-60 Directing health care team members in emergency situations
S-62 Setting priorities
S-65 Applying ethical principles
S-69 Recording devices implanted or explanted during procedures
S-70 Classifying the surgical wound

THE CONCEPT OF COMMUNICATION

Communication is perhaps one of the fundamental examples of a common phenomenon that is described using process-oriented concepts. Concepts are the elements in a set that are grouped together so that each element of the set has diverse characteristics, yet the entire set is classified and referred to by a common name. For example, leaves, petals, stamen, and stem are all elements of a set that are often commonly referred to as a "flower." However, if the elements that describe the common phenomena are dynamic rather than static in nature, they are usually considered to be "process-oriented" elements. Specifically, communication is a combination of

- conveying information and
- exchanging thoughts and/or feelings.

You may be familiar with the definition of communication that includes "sending" and "receiving" messages. The message that is sent and/or received is the content-oriented concept of communication. An item is considered a content-oriented concept if it refers to something that can be either identified and/or measured as a key component of a process. In any form of communication, a message is both sent and received. It is important to identify that the message sent was the message that was received.

EFFECTIVE COMMUNICATION

As noted, a critical element of effective communication is the relationship of the message sent to that of the message received. It is important in any situation to validate the information received as well as that being sent. This is vital in the perioperative setting. The professional nurse must confirm the messages he/she sends directly to the patient and/or family and significant others. One method of validation is asking the receiver to paraphrase, not simply repeat, in his/her own words what information was received. The nurse (as the sender) can develop a therapeutic relationship with a patient and significant others (the receivers) only when there is effective communication between both parties. Effective communication means that any and all messages are

- sent in a manner that is perceived by the receiver as helpful to his/her knowledge deficit and
- perceived by the receiver as helpful to the outcome of his/her care.

There are three basic styles of messages, which appear to be developmentally ordered from least to most effective in meeting situation demands.

- Expressive messages—These are straightforward expressions of the speaker's thoughts and feelings with little or no regard for the situation. The receiver does not usually perceive these types of messages as supportive.

- Conventional messages—These types of messages are deliberately organized to get a specific response from the receiver. Although these messages are appropriate and understood by the receiver, the sender may not be perceived as genuine unless this style of message is always used and not simply used to gain the receiver's support.

- Rhetorical messages—these are elaborate and effective ways to encode the message to be transmitted. These messages are supportive in nature and manage supportive interactions.

Principles of Communication in the Perioperative Setting

The perioperative environment is unique. Perioperative nurses care for patients on a short-term, one-to-one basis in a highly technical environment. Now more than ever, the perioperative nurse must demonstrate effective communication skills with the patient and the family and/or significant others throughout all phases of the patient's surgical journey. To practice these skills, the nurse must identify the factual information that is necessary for the patient and his/her significant others to make intelligent and informed decisions, convey this information accurately, and validate that the appropriate message was received. Using "common sense" principles of communication, and also nursing knowledge, helps to ensure that the majority of the interactions will not only be effective, but logical, systematic, and efficient as well. In order to practice responsible communication in a highly complex and fast-paced perioperative environment, the professional nurse should consider the following.

- Recognize that the patient or clinical situation determines the appropriate chain of communication. For example, if an urgent patient care situation arises, the perioperative nurse will use electronic means of communication, such as the telephone, intercom, or pager so that he/she can remain with the patient. If a clinical situation, such as an equipment malfunction, arises, the nurse often will use human resources, such as notifying the appropriate personnel or delegating non-nursing activities to other personnel while resolving the problem at hand him/herself.

- Refer to facility policies/procedures/protocols and use them as problem-solving tools for patient care or clinical situations. In the patient care or clinical situation examples cited above, the professional nurse combines his/her nursing knowledge with the knowledge of the facility policies and procedures for specific interventions that are initiated on behalf of the patient.

- Practice effective documentation. Comprehensive documentation also is a vital tool in effectively communicating patient care and/or clinical situations. Perioperative documentation is essential for the continuity of care and in the determination of patient outcomes.

COMMUNICATION AS AN INTEGRATED PERIOPERATIVE NURSING PRACTICE BEHAVIOR

The entire process of communication as a method of problem solving occurs during every nurse/patient interaction. As information is encoded, or converted into messages, and then transmitted, the receiver decodes the messages, or determines their meaning. As messages are continuously sent and received, the sender and receiver also use words and gestures, which may have a significant impact on the encoding and decoding. This may even hold true in the intraoperative phase, where the patient may be in various states of analgesia and anesthesia, be visually handicapped, or simply be overwhelmed by the environment. The words and gestures may take on even greater significance as the patient decodes the information received. In addition, there are many other patient considerations on any given day that affect communication, such as physical limitations; psychological, physical, or psychosocial stressors; anger; fear, anxiety, or panic; impairment of perception; unrealistic or inadequate self-concept; and faulty communication skills.

Cultural Diversity Considerations

Today, more than ever, knowledge of cultural diversity issues is imperative at all levels of nursing practice. Every patient must be evaluated for individual cultural differences. Cultural considerations in the perioperative setting, such as the use of blood products, organ transplant, and disposal of body parts to name only a few, often arise because of the increasing number of multicultural patients. These considerations often increase the stress associated with the already stressful situation of needing surgery, experienced by patients who may not be able to communicate with their health care providers. The perioperative nurse must respect all patients' beliefs and faith, and also be perceptive of and sensitive to their communication issues. The patient's value system, ethnicity, and culture must be respected and incorporated into the perioperative plan of care. Some examples of the cultural differences in beliefs regarding health care are as follows.

- Vietnamese—Many perceive illness and suffering as an inevitable part of life. In addition, some also believe that one's longevity is predetermined, therefore, care that saves or prolongs life is pointless. Many Vietnamese also believe that surgery disturbs the soul or causes the spirit to leave the body.
- Hindu—Hindus perceive that blood and semen are life-giving forces, which should not be wasted. Therefore, they may be reluctant to give blood for laboratory tests or donations. Hindus prefer to die at home.
- Moslem—Moslems are against organ donation, cremation, and postmortem examinations. Moslems practice daylight fasting during the month of Ramadan, which varies every year. During this fast, they may refuse medications or injections. Additionally, Moslems prefer that the health care provider is the same gender as the patient.

Because of the demands on nurses' time in today's health care environment, it is unrealistic to expect that nurses will be able to learn all of the pertinent cultural and health aspects of every culture. There are, however, some simple measure nurses can take to provide culturally responsible care, such as,

- recognizing that beliefs and values vary not only between different cultures, but also within cultures;
- regarding the values and beliefs of different cultures, not only within the health care context, but also historically, spiritually, and religiously;
- being conscious of their own cultural values as well as biases;
- attempting to understand the nonverbal communications of their own and other cultures (eg, body language, personal space preferences);
- being aware of interpretation services in their health care facilities; and
- stocking pretranslated materials.

Confidentiality

One of the most basic patient's rights is that of privacy. Confidentiality of patient information is a primary component of patient privacy. It is imperative that the perioperative nurse protect the patient from unwarranted invasions of privacy.

Today, increasing attention is being given to the privacy of medical information largely due to the new provisions of the Health Insurance Portability and Accountability Act (HIPAA) as promulgated by the United States Department of Health and Human Services (HHS), which includes regulations for the protection of patient privacy and the management of individual health information. The HIPAA legislation was passed on August 21, 1996. Prior to this enactment, there were only fragmented laws that allowed health information to be disseminated without notice or consent for reasons other than medical treatment or reimbursement. The major components of the law include

- standards for electronic transactions;
- a national, unique identifier for health care providers and employers;
- standards for privacy of individually identifiably health care information; and
- standards for the security of all forms of identifiable health care information.

Maintaining the privacy and confidentiality of the patient's sensitive health care data has always been an integral part of nursing practice. Perioperative nurses must understand the sensitivity of their communications with all members of the health care team and take the necessary measures to protect patient privacy at all times.

Types of Communication

Taking all of the factors discussed above into consideration, it is therefore vitally important that the professional nurse integrate the various types of communication into perioperative nursing practice.

- Verbal Communication—this is described as the use of words and various elements of language.
  - Denotative meaning—this refers to the meaning that is shared by individuals who use a common language. For example, members of the surgical team understand the concrete meaning of terms such as *scalpel* and *skin prep*. Denotatively, communicating to the patient's family or significant others that the patient's condition is "serious" describes a condition that is potentially threatening to the patient's well-being or life.
  - Connotative meaning—this is the meaning that a word assumes separately from what it explicitly describes. Connotatively, telling the patient's family or significant others that the patient's condition is "serious" implies concern and a sympathetic attitude toward both the patient and his/her significant others.
  - Diction—this is defined as the sender's choice of words or grammar, which will always influence the nature of any verbal communication. It is critical that the nurse communicate with the patient, family, and significant others in words they can understand. For example, it is better to ask a patient, "When was the last time you had anything to eat or drink?" instead of "Have you been NPO since midnight?"
  - Pacing—this is defined as the speed at which a message is delivered. Verbal communication is more successful when the message is delivered calmly at a slow speed. This is especially true when communicating with patients who are anxious or sedated.
  - Intonation—this refers to the tone of voice in which a message is stated. A message may be stated simply, but how it is stated and in what tone of voice may convey something different, such as interest, alarm, indifference, or annoyance.
  - Clarity or brevity—these describe communication that is clear, simple, short, and to the point. Encoding information into short, simple words and using real life experiences to support the messages helps to establish the nurse as a therapeutic and credible resource for the patient, family, and significant others.
- Nonverbal Communication—this is defined as behaviors that are used either consciously or unconsciously by the sender, which the receiver decodes with the message and uses to determine the reliability of the message. The major components of nonverbal communication include the following.
  - General appearance of the sender, including physical condition, dress, grooming, posture, facial expression, and eye contact.
  - Emotional responses of the sender to the receiver's questions or comments.
  - Hand movements of the sender in relation to the message, such as closed fists, open palms, moving toward the receiver, tapping, or fidgeting.
  - Touch, either in a nontherapeutic connotation, or while the therapeutic relationship is being established, must be used with discretion. Historically, touch has been a part of the healing concept. The use of touch, however, also can be associated with unacceptable social behavior, is against certain cultural norms, and may simply be perceived as more annoying then helpful to some patients. Therefore, the nurse must assess the patient's desire or need for touch before it is offered as a therapeutic modality.
  - Closing in on the patient's personal space, or intimate zone (ie, within 18 inches or less from the body). Nurses often must perform interventions within this space. Nonverbal behaviors that demonstrate a high level of empathy while working within this zone are helpful, including eye contact, moderate gesturing, and leaning toward rather than away from the patient.
- Metacommunication—this is defined as the relationship aspect of communication and includes "reading between the lines" or going beyond the surface content of the message to the distinctions

of its meaning. This is an important consideration when interacting with pediatric patients. If a child perceives a conflict between the verbal and nonverbal messages, the child's trust in the nurse as caregiver will be diminished. For example, if the nurse asks a child if it is "OK" to give him/her an injection, the child replies "No," and receives the shot anyway, it is unlikely that this nurse will be able to establish and maintain a therapeutic relationship with this child.

INFORMATION TO BE COMMUNICATED TO PATIENTS/ FAMILY/SIGNIFICANT OTHERS

As recipients of care, all patients are entitled to the assurance of quality health care, privacy, confidentiality, and personal dignity. The delivery of patient-centered care is guided by inherent ethical, legal, and moral principles. Therefore, these principles serve as the foundation for perioperative care and are crucial to achieving positive patient outcomes. According to AORN's "Perioperative Patient Outcomes," behavioral response is considered one of the four domains of the perioperative patient focused model of care, along with physiological responses, patient safety, and the health system. Each domain represents specific phenomena of concern to the perioperative nurse and the needs of the patient and his/her family. Communication plays an integral role in the delivery of care according to the rights and principles described above, but especially as it relates to the behavioral responses of the patient and his/her family or significant others.

Examples of patient outcomes in this domain include the following.

- The patient demonstrates knowledge of expected responses to the operative or invasive procedures.
- The patient demonstrates knowledge of nutritional requirements related to the operative or other invasive procedure.
- The patient demonstrates knowledge of pain management.
- The patient participates in decisions affecting his or her perioperative plan of care.
- The patient's care is consistent with the perioperative plan of care.
- The patient's right to privacy is maintained.
- The patient is the recipient of competent and ethical care within legal standards of practice.
- The patient's value system, lifestyle, ethnicity, and culture are considered, respected, and incorporated in the perioperative plan of care.

In order for the patient to achieve the outcomes listed above, it is imperative that the communication between the perioperative nurse and the patient is effective. This communication is only effective if the nurse (ie, sender) is aware of the principles of communication and uses the requisite skills to establish and maintain a therapeutic relationship so that the patient (ie, receiver) perceives that the information is useful. Therefore, the combination of nursing knowledge and communication skills facilitates the development of the therapeutic relationship and the attainment of optimal patient outcomes.

Consistent with the patient outcome standards listed above, but dependent upon the patient's physical and psychological status, the following information must be communicated between the nurse and the patient and his/her family.

- Verification of the operative procedure—The patient must confirm, either by an oral statement or in writing on the consent form, the type of procedure they are scheduled to undergo.
- The sequence of events and expectations during each phase of the patient's perioperative experience—The patient needs information regarding the sequence of events for the surgical and recovery processes related to his planned operative or invasive procedure. This information also is communicated to the family/significant others according to the patient's preference. The patient should be allowed to ask questions, accurately describe the sequence of events, repeat instructions correctly, and verbalize satisfaction with the content and process of the communication.
- Expected responses and outcomes—The patient must be informed of the outcomes and responses to the operative and/or invasive procedure in realistic terms. A patient may have had prior experiences with surgery—positive or negative—or know someone who had a similar procedure with reportedly negative outcomes. In today's variety of procedural settings and with the emphasis on early discharge, while the patient may state the outcome expectations for his/her

procedure, the communication may not support his/her statements. For example, the patient who asks, "Will I really go home this afternoon?" may be metacommunicating the need for reassurance. It also is important for the perioperative nurse to recognize that information often determines the patient's attitude for the duration of their perioperative course and can affect the expected outcomes.

- The patient's attitudes and feelings about the perioperative experience, taking into consideration the patient's ethnicity and cultural beliefs— The manner in which something is said is as important as what is actually said. Equally important for the nurse to remember is that listening is an active process, and it must be practiced as such when the patient and significant others share their feelings about the impending surgical or invasive procedure. Listening is a skill that demands focusing, questioning, and validation as well as time to process the information received. If the listener is judging the sender or the message, or is distracted or preparing a response in advance, he/she is not listening effectively or gaining all the information possible from the communication. Interference and noise, which are commonplace in most perioperative settings, also can negatively affect listening and consequently distort the message. The perioperative nurse also must verify that the patient is internalizing his/her communications by repeatedly affirming the role of advocate and encouraging the patient and significant others to express their feelings.

The professional perioperative nurse realizes that he/she performs a special role as the patient's advocate in a strange and often frightening environment. The nurse's primary goal is to establish rapport with the patient and his/her significant others, which will help him/her establish and maintain a meaningful and therapeutic relationship with the patient. The relationship should include and respect the attitudes, behaviors, feelings, and culture of the patient and significant others. Therefore, the following aspects of communication are especially vital during each phase of the patient's surgical experience:

Preoperative Nursing Considerations

Nursing considerations in the preoperative phase highlight the establishment of rapport with the patient and significant others. Key elements in this phase include, but are not limited to,

- assessing the knowledge base of the patient and family/significant others;
- assessing the relationship between the patient and significant others;
- maintaining awareness of the verbal, nonverbal, and metacommunication styles; and
- soliciting underlying concerns or issues regarding the procedure or risk for anesthesia that must be communicated to other members of the surgical team.

AORN statements of competency related to the preoperative nursing considerations include the competency to

- assess the physiological health status of the patient;
- assess the psychosocial health status of the patient/family;
- formulate nursing diagnosis based on health status data;
- establish patient goals based on nursing diagnosis;
- develop a plan of care that prescribes nursing actions to achieve patient goals; and
- participate in patient/family teaching.

Intraoperative Nursing Considerations

The intraoperative phase is often the one that causes the most stress for the patient's family. Therefore, intraoperative nursing considerations emphasize helping both the patient and family/significant others cope with the natural and unnatural stress and anxiety associated with the operative or invasive procedure. A key consideration during this phase is the coordination of communication between the various members of the surgical team and the patient's family/significant others. Relevant AORN statements of competency for communication during the intraoperative phase include the competency to

- develop a plan of care that prescribes nursing actions to achieve patient goals;
- implement nursing actions in transferring the patient according to the prescribed plan;

- participate in patient/family teaching;
- respect patient's rights;
- perform nursing actions that demonstrate accountability; and
- continually reassess all components of patient care based on new data.

Postoperative Nursing Considerations

Postoperative nursing communication begins with the communication of all pertinent data regarding the preoperative and intraoperative phases of care to the nurse in the receiving unit (ie, PACU, ICU, step-down area, medical-surgical unit). The emphasis in this phase is the effective use of communication skills to promote a satisfactory recovery from the surgical or invasive procedure and also the associated anesthesia or sedation. AORN statements of competency for communication in the postoperative phase include the competency to

- evaluate patient outcomes;
- measure effectiveness of nursing care; and
- continuously reassess all components of patient care based on new data.

SUMMARY

Providing quality health care to patients in the perioperative setting is a complex process that requires a wide range of knowledge, skills, and collaborative efforts. This multidisciplinary process requires the use of effective communication skills throughout all phases of the patient's perioperative experience and must include the patient's family and/or significant others. In today's health care environment, communication is much more than simply carrying on a conversation with or imparting information to others. Therefore, nurses must be aware of their own communication skills and individual competencies.

Just as the practice of nursing is both art and science, so is the practice of effective communication. The situational context of communication takes on greater significance for the perioperative nurse. Effective communication skills must be developed, mastered, and used resourcefully to promote positive outcomes for both the patient and his/her family and significant others.

CASE STUDIES

Case Study: Ms. N

Ms. N is a 43-year-old Vietnamese immigrant who is admitted to your ambulatory surgery center for a right breast biopsy. Upon admission, she is accompanied by her husband and 80-year-old mother. She speaks English fairly well and is able to understand your introduction and explanations. During the initial assessment, she is sitting in the chair with her arms folded and makes limited eye contact with you. She and her mother are speaking in Vietnamese throughout your assessment, and at one point, her mother gets up and walks out of the room. After which, Ms. N begins to cry, tells you that she wants to cancel the surgery, and asks you to tell the surgeon as she prepares to leave.

Points to Consider

Some key principles of communication and cultural considerations in this scenario include

- nonverbal communication—sitting with arms folded, lack of eye contact, crying;
- verbal message—she wants to cancel the surgery; and
- cultural considerations—recognition that she may view the breast mass as something that is inevitable and that the surgery may be futile and also upset her soul/spirit.

Appropriate nursing considerations and interventions for Ms. N would include

- recognizing her cultural beliefs and values;
- regarding her cultural, spiritual, and religious values and beliefs;
- being conscious of your own cultural values and biases;
- attempting to understand her nonverbal communications;
- assessing the knowledge base of Ms. N and her family;
- assessing the relationship between Ms. N and her family; and
- maintaining awareness of the verbal, nonverbal, and metacommunication styles.

Case Study: Mr. J

Mr. J is your 52-year-old neighbor who has just been transported to the preoperative holding area. He is scheduled for a colon resection and has requested that you be his circulating nurse. You are visiting him in the holding area and reviewing his chart. As you are standing there, he looks at you, lifts himself up toward you, touches your forearm, and asks you, "Be sure to let my girlfriend in the waiting area know how I am doing and if the cancer has spread to my liver, since the doctor told me it might have already."

Points to Consider

Some key principles of communication and perioperative nursing considerations in this scenario include

- verbal communication—"Be sure to let my girlfriend know if the cancer has spread to my liver, since the doctor told me it might have already.";
- nonverbal communication—eye contact, moving toward you, touch;
- metacommunication—concern, possibly fear or anxiety;
- verification of the operative procedure—either orally or in writing on the consent form;
- the sequence of events and expectations during Mr. J's perioperative experience;
- realistic expected responses and outcomes to the procedure; and
- Mr. J's right to privacy.

SUGGESTED LEARNING ACTIVITIES

- ◆ Attempt to answer the following questions about the demographics of your facility.
    - What are the most common ethnic groups seen at your facility?
    - What do you know about these groups of people?
    - What are the beliefs held by these groups that could effect the delivery of care during surgery?
    - How might you alter your approach and communication to patients from these groups to facilitate their care?
- ◆ Are there certain situations that present difficulties or patients with whom you find it difficult to communicate? What do you imagine limits your communication skills in these situations? What could you do to enhance your skills?
- ◆ Review what services are provided by your facility to deal with patients who are not able to speak English. How do you arrange for these services?
- ◆ Do you hold any personal beliefs that inhibit your communication skills with patients? What could you do to improve?
- ◆ Seek out a peer who you respect for his or her communication abilities and ask for input about dealing with communication difficulties.

RECOMMENDED STUDY MATERIALS

AORN, "ANA code for nurses with interpretive statements—Explications for perioperative nursing," in *Standards, Recommended Practices, and Guidelines* (Denver: AORN, Inc, 2002) 53-70.

AORN, "Competency statements in perioperative nursing," in *Standards, Recommended Practices, and Guidelines* (Denver: AORN, Inc, 2002) 19-21.

AORN, "Recommended practices for documentation of perioperative nursing care," in *Standards, Recommended Practices, and Guidelines* (Denver: AORN, Inc, 2002) 217-219.

AORN, "Standards: Patient Outcomes," in *Standards, Recommended Practices, and Guidelines* (Denver: AORN, Inc, 2002) 173-182.

ASPAN, *Standards of Perianesthesia Nursing Practice* (Cherry Hill, NJ: American Society of PeriAnesthesia Nurses, 2000).

Bush, K, "Do you really listen to patients?" *RN* 64 (March 2001) 35-37.

Calvin, R; Kolar, K R, "Development of a family liaison model during operative procedures," *AORN Journal* 72 (August 2000) 308, 310.

Carelock, J; Innerarity, S, "Critical incidents: Effective communication and documentation," *Critical Care Nursing Quarterly* 23 (February 2001) 59-66.

Downes, M, "False cultural assumptions: A bar to effective communication," *Nursing Times* 95 (August 1999) 42-43.

Dreger, V; Tremback, T, "Optimize patient health by treating literacy and language barriers," *AORN Journal* 75 (February 2002) 280-283.

Elliott, R; Wright, L, "Verbal communication: What do critical care nurses say to their unconscious or sedated patients?" *Journal of Advanced Nursing* 29 (June 1999) 1412-1420.

Ellis, J R; Hartley, C L, *Nursing in Today's*

World: Challenges, Issues, and Trends, sixth ed (Philadelphia: Lippincott Raven, 1998).

Guild, R, "Effective communication," *Journal of Community Nursing* 9 (September 1995) 10, 12, 14.

Ide, P; Fleming, C, "A successful practice model for the OR," *AORN Journal* 70 (November 1999) 811, 813.

Martin, G W, "Communication breakdown or ideal speech situation: The problem of nurse advocacy," *Nursing Ethics: An International Journal for Health Care Professionals* 5 (March 1998) 147-157.

Naish, J, "The route to effective nurse-patient communication," *Nursing Times* 92 (April 1996) 24-30.

Petersen, C, "How private is private? HIPAA," *SSM* 7 (December 2001) 49-51.

Reilly, C E; Lambrecht, M E, "The cognitive model: Interventions for improved patient-provider communication," *Journal of Psychosocial Nursing & Mental Health Services* 39 (June 2001) 32-39; 48-49.

Sullivan, A, "Viewpoint: Culture speaks louder than words," *SSM* 7 (June 2001) 10-13.

Sullivan, N; Swenson, J, "Creating a healing environment in the surgery department," *Surgical Services Management* 4 (December 1998) 25-28.

Summers, L C, "Mutual timing: An essential component of provider/patient communication," *Journal of the American Academy of Nurse Practitioners* 14 (January 2002) 19-25.

Swanson, E, et al, "An application of an effective interdisciplinary health-focused cross-cultural collaboration," *Journal of Professional Nursing* 17 (January/February 2001) 33-39.

Sweetland, J L, "Therapeutic touch in traditional settings," *Surgical Services Management* 4 (December 1998) 30-34.

Thiederman, S, "Improving communication in a diverse health care environment: As many as 20 languages may be encountered among the staff and patients of a health care facility," *Healthcare Financial Management* 50 (November 1996) 74-75.

Usher, K; Monkley, D, "Effective communication in an intensive care setting: Nurses' stories," *Contemporary Nurse* 10 (March 2001) 91-101.

Williams, C A; Gossett, M T, "Nursing communication: Advocacy for the patient or physician?" *Clinical Nursing Research* 10 (August 2001) 332-340.

Wright, F; Cohen, S; Caroselli, C, "Diverse decisions: How culture affects decision making," *Critical Care Nursing Clinics of North America* 9 (March 1997) 63-74.

CHAPTER 13: PARTICIPATE IN DISCHARGE PLANNING

Sylvia Durrance, RN, BSN, CNOR

Perioperative nurses' responsibilities in discharge planning have increased with the increase in outpatient surgeries, reduced length of hospital stays, and emphasis on self-care. The perioperative nurse may be the only nursing contact for many patients undergoing operative and invasive procedures. This chapter provides the perioperative nurse with information for use in creating a multi-disciplinary discharge plan. The emphasis is on specific perioperative nursing activities.

The nurse must consider educational assessment (ie, what the patient needs and wants to know), patient readiness to learn and barriers to learning, level and types of information to be provided, and family participation. The perioperative nurse also must be cognizant of the multiple sociocultural influences that contribute to the patient's and family's attitude toward health care, coping strategies, and compliance with postoperative requirements. Perioperative discharge planning requires the perioperative nurse to have an understanding of

- the nursing process;
- the philosophy, definition, and scope of perioperative nursing practice;
- AORN perioperative nursing competencies;
- standards of perioperative clinical practice;
- perioperative patient outcomes;
- pediatric, adolescent, adult, and geriatric teaching/learning principles;
- roles and functions of the multidisciplinary health care team; and
- available community resources.

Perioperative nurses must be able to interpret, synthesize, and apply the above information in specific patient situations. This chapter reviews the required knowledge and skills. Opportunities are provided to apply these skills to case study situations and specified learning activities. A bibliography lists recommended sources for independent study.

LEARNING OBJECTIVES

Perioperative nurses preparing for the CNOR exam should obtain the areas of knowledge and skill required for discharge planning. At the completion of this chapter, the applicant should be able to:

1. Discuss discharge planning activities and rationales and apply them in specific clinical settings.
2. Use assessment data to develop an appropriate discharge plan in collaboration with patient, family, and a multidisciplinary health care team.
3. Assess patients' and families' readiness to learn status.
4. Evaluate patients' and families' understanding of the plan.
5. Evaluate the plan's effectiveness.
6. Identify need for patient referral to other health care team members, such as social workers or home health professionals, or nurse collaboration with extended care facility nurses.

TASK STATEMENT; AREAS OF KNOWLEDGE AND SKILL

Task Statement

Participate in the collaborative discharge planning process to optimize postoperative health status.

Areas of Knowledge

K-1 Health assessment techniques
K-2 Anatomy and physiology
K-3 Pathophysiology
K-4 Pharmacology and anesthetic agents
K-5 Pain management
K-6 Principles of wound healing
K-7 Diagnostic procedures and results
K-8 Preoperative patient preparation activities
K-9 Surgical, anesthetic, and other perioperative interventions
K-10 Expected outcomes related to identified interventions
K-11 Physiologic responses to the surgical experience
K-15 Risks for injury, including but not limited to, skin, positioning, and retained foreign body
K-17 Postoperative complications
K-20 Sociology (eg, cultural and ethnic influences, family patterns, spirituality and related practices)
K-21 Communication theories and techniques
K-22 Behavioral responses to the surgical experience
K-23 Discharge planning
K-24 Theories of and resources for patient/family education
K-25 *Perioperative Nursing Data Set* (PNDS)
K-27 Microbiology and infection control
K-28 Standard and transmission-based precautions
K-30 Interventions to optimize safety
K-37 Principles of product evaluation, cost-containment, and resource management
K-39 Patient rights and responsibilities
K-40 Legal responsibilities and implications for patient care
K-41 Approved nursing diagnoses (eg, NANDA)
K-42 Nursing research and evidence-based practice
K-44 Regulatory standards and voluntary guidelines
K-45 AORN *Standards, Recommended Practices, and Guidelines*
K-46 AORN position statements (eg, bloodborne pathogens, do-not-resuscitate orders [DNR])
K-47 Principles of problem solving
K-48 Quality improvement principles
K-50 Defining characteristics of impaired individuals (eg, substance abuse, psychological disturbance, compromised performance)
K-52 Defining characteristics of domestic abuse (eg, child, elder, partner/spouse)
K-53 Rules, responsibilities, and duties of health care team members and internal and external support service personnel
K-56 Implants (eg, handling, tracking, sterilization)

Areas of Skill

S-1 Confirming patient identity, operative site, and procedure
S-2 Collecting, analyzing, and prioritizing patient data
S-3 Using health assessment techniques (eg, interview, observation, auscultation, palpation, percussion)
S-4 Communicating effectively (verbal and nonverbal)
S-5 Advocating and protecting patient rights
S-6 Evaluating environment for discharge care
S-7 Assessing and managing pain
S-8 Assessing for potential abuse (eg, substance, domestic)
S-9 Assessing readiness to learn, knowledge level, and preferred learning style
S-10 Identifying barriers to learning
S-11 Identifying risk of infection and injury
S-12 Identifying cultural, spiritual, and ethnic issues in care
S-13 Identifying age specific needs
S-14 Formulating a nursing diagnosis
S-15 Collaborating with other members on the health care team
S-16 Applying AORN *Standards, Recommended Practices, and Guidelines*
S-17 Applying the *Perioperative Nursing Data Set* (PNDS)
S-18 Delineating and communicating measurable patient outcomes
S-19 Participating in quality improvement activities
S-20 Maintaining accurate patient records
S-23 Applying regulatory standards and voluntary guidelines
S-24 Developing a patient and family education plan
S-26 Incorporating community and institutional resources into plan of care
S-27 Delegating interventions and/or assigning tasks
S-28 Adapting to changing situations and technologies
S-29 Performing nursing interventions
S-33 Anticipating the needs for equipment, supplies, and personnel
S-35 Maintaining the dignity, modesty, and privacy of the patient and protecting the confidentiality of patient information

S-36 Applying principles of aseptic technique and infection control
S-46 Anticipating and evaluating the effects of pharmacological and anesthetic agents
S-48 Detecting significant changes in the environment
S-50 Adapting to special and unusual needs
S-51 Identifying and communicating changes in patient status
S-52 Documenting nursing interventions and patient response
S-56 Measuring, evaluating, and documenting patient outcomes
S-62 Setting priorities
S-65 Applying ethical principles
S-67 Evaluating for signs and symptoms of injury
S-70 Classifying the surgical wound

PREOPERATIVE NURSING ACTIVITIES

The purpose of a discharge plan is to prepare to move the patient from one level of care to the next with the overall goal of return to the optimum achievable level of function. The patient may be discharged to home, a rehabilitation facility, or other identified location to recover from the intervention. The plan reflects desired patient outcomes and is developed collaboratively by the patient, family, significant other(s), and members of the health care team.

Discharge planning actually begins in the physician's office when the patient first makes the decision to undergo an invasive procedure. For this reason, it is imperative that the perioperative nurse reviews the chart entries by other members of the health care team; this also ensures that appropriate documentation is present. Discharge planning is a component of the care delivered throughout the admission period.

Preoperative nursing activities that contribute to the discharge plan may include:

- ◆ Chart review—Required documentation includes:
  - History and physical examination within regulatory required time frame
  - Laboratory diagnostic data
  - Signed operative consent
  - Advanced directive education
  - Physician documentation of informed consent
  - Verification of site and side of procedure

- ◆ Patient/family interview
  - Verify documented assessment data.
  - Collect any undocumented information.
  - Assess level of understanding of and attitude toward the scheduled procedure.
  - Assess ability and motivation to follow instructions:
    - o Age
    - o Educational level
    - o Ethnicity
    - o Language
    - o Socio-cultural status
    - o Anxiety level
    - o Acceptance of diagnosis and planned procedure
    - o Level of alertness and orientation
    - o Language and reading level of print media
    - o Level of satisfaction with care received

- ◆ Participation in development and implementation of the discharge plan.
  - Contribute assessment data.
  - Actively listen during the preoperative interview to determine concerns not openly expressed.
  - Ask open-ended questions.
  - Encourage patient, family, and significant other participation.
    - o Give them the opportunity to ask questions regarding any concerns.
    - o Patients and families interact with health care providers at multiple access points. Expressions of concern and questions regarding the planned procedure are affected by the cultural knowledge level and communication skills of the provider. It is well within the scope of the perioperative nurse to elicit further information that can affect postoperative care.

- ◆ Communicate perioperative information to appropriate team members.
  - *Example*—A patient tells the perioperative nurse that she has been taking herbal medication to relieve her depression. The nurse knows that some herbal medications for depression may interact with anesthetic agents and immediately communicates this information to the anesthesia care provider. Begin the discharge planning by:
    - o Encouraging her to express what makes her feel she needs the herbs for depression. By giving the nurse this information, she has offered an opening to discuss issues that the nurse may be able to either assist with or direct her to further resources.

- o Explaining to the patient that herbs are real medications with real actions, and that she should always communicate this information to anyone who cares for her.

INTRAOPERATIVE NURSING ACTIVITIES

During the intraoperative phase, the perioperative nurse continually assesses the patient and adjusts the nursing plan based on the patient's physiological and psychological responses. The data that is collected intraoperatively contributes to the discharge plan.

- ◆ The nurse is knowledgeable regarding the planned intervention and anesthesia care and the expected postoperative outcomes related to the surgical procedure.
  - *Example*—A patient is scheduled for a femoral popliteal bypass. The nurse knows that the patient must be educated in wound care, infection control, and methods to assist in preventing further disease progress (eg, elimination of smoking, low cholesterol diet). This information will be part of the postoperative discharge plan.

- ◆ The nurse is aware and understands the implications of intraoperative unplanned events or complications that might affect the patient's postoperative outcomes and communicates them to appropriate members of the team.
  - *Example*—A patient experiences a reaction to a medication intraoperatively. The nurse must ensure that this reaction is entered into the patient record and communicated to the postoperative care team to prevent further injury.
  - *Example*—A patient demonstrates a break in skin integrity related to the electrosurgical dispersive pad. The nurse documents this event and communicates with other team members to arrange for postoperative follow-up.
  - *Example*—The nurse notes an unexpected amount of drainage in the pleurevac immediately following a thoracotomy and immediately alerts the surgeon. The wound is reopened and bleeding is controlled before leaving the OR.

POSTOPERATIVE NURSING ACTIVITIES

The nurse verifies and implements the discharge plan following an invasive procedure. The plan must meet the expectations of a multidisciplinary health care team. The 2001 *Comprehensive Accreditation Manual for Hospitals* of the Joint Commission on Accreditation of Healthcare Organizations (JCAHO) integrated all discharge planning into a multidisciplinary process.

JCAHO Standards require that the patient's medical record includes documentation of

- ◆ initial assessment and continual reassessments;
- ◆ nursing diagnoses and patient care needs;
- ◆ interventions identified to meet the patient's nursing care needs;
- ◆ the nursing care provided and the involvement of the patient, family, physicians, nurses, social workers, and other professionals as appropriate;
- ◆ arrangements made for services required after discharge;
- ◆ exchange of appropriate patient care and clinical information when patients are admitted, referred, transferred, or discharged;
- ◆ the patient's response to, and the outcomes of, care provided;
- ◆ abilities of the patient and/or significant other(s) to manage continuing care needs post discharge;
- ◆ a discharge summary and instructions forwarded to the primary care practitioner; and
- ◆ follow-up assessment and clarification of discharge.

In addition, AORN has developed "Outcome Standards: Perioperative Patient Outcomes," which were revised in 2001 to incorporate AORN's *Perioperative Nursing Data Set* (PNDS). These standards reflect the responsibility of the perioperative nurse to focus on patient outcomes in planning nursing interventions to help surgical patients achieve the highest attainable outcome through the perioperative experience.[8]

- ◆ Participate in evaluating the nursing care plan. The following outcome standards are from the 2002 edition of the PNDS and should be considered in the evaluation of all patients.

  Domain: Perioperative Safety
  - The patient is free from signs and symptoms

of injury caused by extraneous objects. (O2)

- The patient is free of signs and symptoms of chemical injury. (O3)
- The patient is free of signs and symptoms of electrical injury. (O4)
- The patient is free of signs and symptoms of injury related to positioning. (O5)
- The patient is free from signs and symptoms of laser injury. (O6)
- The patient is free of signs and symptoms radiation injury. (O7)
- The patient is free of signs and symptoms of injury related to transfer/transport. (O8)
- The patient receives appropriate medication(s), safely administered during the perioperative period. (O9)

Domain: Physiologic Responses

- The patient is free of signs and symptoms of infection. (O10)
- The patient has wound/tissue perfusion consistent with or improved from baseline levels established preoperatively. (011)
- The patient's fluid, electrolyte, and acid-base balances are consistent with or improved from baseline levels established preoperatively. (013)
- The patient's respiratory function is consistent with or improved from baseline levels established preoperatively. (014)
- The patient's cardiovascular function is consistent with or improved from baseline levels established preoperatively. (015)
- The patient demonstrates and/or reports adequate pain control throughout the perioperative period. (029)
- The patient's neurological function is consistent with or improved from baseline levels established preoperatively. (030)

Domain: Behavioral Responses—Patient and Family

- The patient demonstrates knowledge of expected responses to the operative or invasive procedure. (031)
- The patient demonstrates knowledge of nutritional requirements related to the operative or other invasive procedure. (018)
- The patient demonstrates knowledge of medication management. (019)
- The patient demonstrates knowledge of pain management. (020)
- The patient participates in the rehabilitation process. (021).
- The patient demonstrates knowledge of wound healing. (022)
- The patient participates in decisions affecting his or her perioperative plan of care. (023)
- The patient's care is consistent with the perioperative plan of care. (024)
- The patient's right to privacy is maintained. (025)
- The patient is the recipient of competent and ethical care within legal standards of practice. (026).
- The patient receives consistent and comparable care regardless of the setting. (027)
- The patient's value system, lifestyle, ethnicity, and culture are considered, respected, and incorporated in the perioperative plan of care. (028)

◆ The perioperative nurse contributes to discharge planning by applying and communicating intraoperative data.
  - *Example*—A patient is undergoing a low anterior resection for adenocarcinoma of the rectum. The unit nurse has begun a discharge plan incorporating the care plan for abdominal surgery. The tumor is determined to be more extensive than planned, and the patient has a colostomy rather than the planned anastamosis. The perioperative nurse identifies the need for the patient to learn stomal care. She communicates with the case manager to arrange consultation with the enterostomal therapist and a home health nurse.

◆ The perioperative nurse contributes to discharge planning through communication of appropriate information to the patient and family.
  - *Example*—The nurse is preparing for the discharge of a 74-year-old woman who has undergone an AV fistula in preparation for dialysis. The patient and her family express concerns that they will have difficulty getting the patient to her dialysis appointment three times a week. The nurse assesses their level of understanding of the importance of these visits and provides them with information regarding local resources that provide transportation to elderly patients. Provision of this information is documented, and the nurse makes a referral to the social services department to ensure that the family is able to take advantage of these resources.

SUMMARY

Appropriate discharge planning is a critical component of the perioperative nursing process. Adequate planning ensures that the patient has a successful recovery with minimal complications and is able to return to the optimal achievable level of function. The perioperative nurse is a member of a multidisciplinary team, which may include case management, counseling, physical therapy, education, and home health care. The team works together to return the patient to a satisfactory outcome.

CASE STUDIES

Case Study: Mrs. J

Mrs. J is a 37-year-old housewife and mother of four children (two girls aged 13 and 8 and two boys aged 10 and 4). She was a teacher prior to her marriage. She is scheduled to have a right simple mastectomy with prosthetic reconstruction and a tram flap for post-mastectomy reconstruction of her left breast.

Her husband is a 43-year-old business executive who travels frequently and does not routinely participate in household tasks or child care. They have no nearby relatives and are not active in any church or social groups. Mrs. J expresses concern that there is no one available to manage her household and care for her children while she is recovering. She states that her husband "already has his hands full supporting us without worrying about me."

Points to Consider

- What events, situations, or fears might have an effect on her postoperative course and discharge?
- How will her lifestyle affect her postoperative course and discharge plan?
- What general topics should be included in the discharge plan?
- What specific topics should be included in the discharge plan?
- How would you assess ability and readiness to understand discharge teaching?
- How would you validate understanding?
- How would you include the family in the plan?
- When would you begin planning discharge with Mrs. J?
- What will participation in rehabilitation mean to Mrs. J?
- What is her coping mechanism?

Discussion of Points to Consider

- What events, situations, or fears might have an effect on her postoperative course and discharge?
  - o Family separation
  - o Loss of independence
  - o Worry about child care
  - o Worry about procedure and changes in body image
  - o Worry about postoperative course including pain, drains, wound care, and progressive return to mobility

- How will her lifestyle affect her postoperative course and discharge plan?
  She is worried about her household and her children and does not want to "burden" her husband. This can have a positive impact of causing her to work hard on her rehabilitation. It could have a potential for a negative impact, if she attempts to rush her recovery. The roles in this family are structured so that there is little shared responsibility. The need for the husband to assume additional responsibility and for Mrs. J to be dependent has the potential to lead to role stress and family tension. The perioperative nurse needs to assess the family and make social services referrals if necessary. The nurse should be aware that the American Cancer Society could provide assistance to this family. The family isolation is also an issue here. Mrs. J needs encouragement to develop outside interests.

- What general topics should be included in the discharge plan?
  - o Responses to the surgical procedure
  - o What to look out for, and when to call the physician's office
  - o Who to call when the physician is not available and contact information
  - o Procedures that must be done at home
  - o Level of activity and expected progression
  - o Medications
  - o Community resources

- What specific topics should be included in the discharge plan?
  - o Progressive exercise program
  - o Avoidance of IVs in her left arm in the future
  - o Specific medication, rationale, and frequency
  - o Any dietary recommendations
  - o Symptoms to look for, such as increased pain, swelling, tenderness or drainage, temperature over 100° F, or chills

- o Progressive resumption of household duties
- o Follow-up care and visits
- o Potential use of community resources for household help

- How would you assess ability and readiness to understand discharge teaching?
  Ability can be assessed through the patient's age, education, job skills, and communication abilities. Readiness to learn could be assessed by the patient asking questions or showing interest in self-care. Mrs. J's past position as a teacher is an asset in learning and performing self-care.

- How would you validate understanding?
  Mrs. J's understanding can be validated by return demonstration of wound care and asking her to repeat other information, such as progressive exercise. Written instructions also should be provided.

- How would you include the family in the plan?
  The family should be included in all phases of the discharge plan. They can assist in validating understanding of the discharge plan. If the children accompany her to the hospital, the nurse should assess their level of understanding. Perhaps the 13-year-old could be taught to help with the drain. The nurse should determine whether Mr. J is aware of the Family Medical Leave Act and community resources for in-home assistance.

- When would you begin planning discharge with Mrs. J?
  The plan should begin as soon as she begins the admission process. Discharge planning should be a component of preregistration activities. The nurse may not be present, but should take time to review the information given and received at this visit for further planning.

- What will participation in rehabilitation mean to Mrs. J?
  Active participation in her rehabilitation will allow Mrs. J to return to independently caring for her household and her family.

- What is her coping mechanism?
  Mrs. J is used to independence in caring for her household and family without any outside help and minimal help from her husband. The nurse can encourage return to independence by teaching her how to care for her incisions, empty her drain reservoir, and manage her medication.

Case Study: Mr. K

Mr. K is a 74-year-old retired airline mechanic and widower with insulin dependent diabetes and severe peripheral vascular disease. He is scheduled for an amputation below the right knee after undergoing a femoral-popliteal bypass one month ago.

Mr. K has lived alone in a second floor apartment with no elevator since the death of his wife. He receives social security and a small pension. He has one son from whom he has been estranged for several years. He smokes a pack of cigarettes a day. His only social contacts are his "drinking buddies."

He feels that he will no longer be able to take care of himself and tells the perioperative nurse that now he "will be useless and might as well just give up."

Points to Consider

- What events, situations, or fears might have an effect on his postoperative course and discharge?
- How will his lifestyle affect his postoperative course and discharge plan?
- What general topics should be included in the discharge plan?
- What specific topics should be included in the discharge plan?
- How would you assess ability and readiness to understand discharge teaching?
- How would you validate understanding?
- How would you include the family in the plan?
- When would you begin planning discharge with Mr. K?
- What will participation in rehabilitation mean to Mr. K?
- What is his coping mechanism?

Discussion of Points to Consider

- What events, situations, or fears might have an effect on his postoperative course and discharge?
  - o Loss of independence
  - o Fear of further disease progression
  - o Isolation
  - o Depression

- How will his lifestyle affect his postoperative course and discharge plan?
  Mr. K's continued smoking and drinking would have a negative effect on his disease progression and surgical recovery. He will likely have to move unless he becomes very proficient with his

artificial limb. He will require referral to social services.

- What general topics should be included in the discharge plan?
  - o Expected responses to the surgical procedure
  - o What to look out for, and when to call the physician's office
  - o Who to call when the physician is not available and contact information
  - o Procedures that must be done at home (eg, wound care, drains, medication management, exercises)
  - o Level of activity and expected progression
  - o Medications
  - o Community resources

- What specific topics should be included in the discharge plan?
  - o Progressive exercise program
  - o Use of artificial limb
  - o Specific medication, rationale, and frequency
  - o Diabetic diet
  - o Relation of smoking cessation to condition
  - o Relation of drinking to diabetes
  - o Symptoms to look for, such as increased pain, swelling, tenderness or drainage, temperature over 100° F, or chills
  - o Progressive resumption of activity
  - o Follow-up care and visits

- How would you assess ability and readiness to understand discharge teaching?
  Ability can be assessed through the patient's age, education, job skills, and communication abilities. Readiness to learn could be assessed by the patient asking questions or showing interest in self-care. Mr. K's depression will be a barrier to learning. His past history as a mechanic may be of use in leaning to use and care for his prosthetic limb.

- How would you validate understanding?
  Mr. K's understanding can be validated by return demonstration of wound care and asking him to repeat other information, such as progressive exercise. It is vitally important with this patient to engage him in a discussion of his understanding of the relation between diabetes and peripheral vascular disease. Written instructions also should be provided.

- How would you include the family in the plan?
  It sounds as if Mr. K's only routine contacts are his "drinking buddies." The nurse should engage Mr. K to talk about his son to determine if there is any possibility of reuniting this family. A social work referral is imperative.

- When would you begin planning discharge with Mr. K?
  The plan should begin as soon as he begins the admission process. Discharge planning should be a component of preregistration activities. The nurse may not be present, but should take time to review the information given and received at this visit for further planning.

- What will participation in rehabilitation mean to Mr. K?
  Mr. K will have to be admitted to an extended care facility until his wound is healed and he has been fitted with and learned to use a prosthesis. He could be anxious to be independent again and participate fully in his rehabilitation. He also could sink into depression, based on his comments to the nurse. He will need referral to a mental health worker and a social worker.

- What is his coping mechanism?
  Unfortunately, all of Mr. K's coping mechanisms are unhealthy. His smoking and drinking have contributed to the progression of his disease. How would the nurse engage him in talking about his diabetes and his vascular disease? Does he understand the disease process, and if so how could he be encouraged to modify his lifestyle?

SUGGESTED LEARNING ACTIVITIES

The following learning activities will be of assistance in determining your level of expertise in contributing to the discharge plan.

- ◆ Review the standards of care for your hospital and evaluate a particular patient's achievement of the outcomes in those standards.

- ◆ Discuss discharge plan for the patient you have selected with other members of the health care team. Ask what changes to the plan they would suggest and why.

- ◆ Evaluate your own strengths and areas for opportunity. Validate your assessment by requesting that peers review you.

- ◆ Work with a preceptor or mentor who demonstrates skill in discharge planning.

- Assist in preparing discharge plans for selected patients.
- Review selected items from the recommended study materials at the end of the chapter.
- Spend time with discharge planners in ambulatory care or home health.
- Talk to a social worker or public health nurse to learn about available community resources for patients.
- Prepare an in-service program on discharge planning for colleagues.

RECOMMENDED STUDY MATERIALS

AORN, *Standards, Recommended Practices, and Guidelines* (Denver: AORN, Inc, 2002).

Beyea, S, ed, *Perioperative Nursing Data Set* second ed (Denver: AORN, Inc, 2002).

Fortunato, N H, ed, *Berry & Kohn's Operating Room Technique*, ninth ed (St Louis: Mosby, Inc, 2000).

Meeker, M H; Rothrock, J C, *Alexander's Care of the Patient in Surgery,* 12th ed (St Louis: Mosby, Inc, 2002).

Weissman, M A; Jasovsky, D A, "Discharge Teaching for Today's Times," *RN* 61 (6) (June 1998) 38-40.

REFERENCES

1. AORN, *Standards, Recommended Practices & Guidelines* (Denver: AORN, Inc, 2002).
2. J Cooper, "Teaching patients in post-operative eye care: The demands of day surgery," *Nursing Standard* 13 (12) (1999) 42-46.
3. V J Fox, "Patient Education and Discharge Planning," in *Alexander's Care of the Patient in Surgery,* M H Meeker, J C Rothrock, eds (St Louis: Mosby, Inc, 1999).
4. A Henderson, W Zernike, "A study of the impact of discharge information for surgical patients," *Journal of Advanced Nursing* 35 (3) (2001) 435-441.
5. JCAHO, *Comprehensive Accreditation Manual for Hospitals* (Oakbrook Terrace, Ill: Joint Commission on Accreditation of Healthcare Organizations, 2001).
6. JCAHO, 2001-2002 *Comprehensive Accreditation Manual of Health Care Networks Supplement* (Oakbrook Terrace, Ill: Joint Commission on Accreditation of Healthcare Organizations, 2001).
7. JCAHO, *Critical Access Hospital Standards* (Oakbrook Terrace, Ill: Joint Commission on Accreditation of Healthcare Organizations, 2002).
8. S Beyea, ed, *Perioperative Nursing Data Set* (Denver: AORN, Inc, 2002).
9. C S Ladden, "Concepts Basic to Perioperative Nursing," in *Alexander's Care of the Patient in Surgery,* M H Meeker, J C Rothrock,eds (St Louis: Mosby, Inc, 1999).
10. J C McCloskey, G M Bulechek, eds, *Nursing Interventions and Classifications* (NIC), second ed (St Louis: Mosby, Inc, 1996).
11. R M Tappen, J Muszic, P Kennedy, "Preoperative assessment and discharge planning for older adults undergoing ambulatory surgery," *AORN Journal* 73 (2) (2001) 464, 467, 469-470.

CHAPTER 14: SELECT AND USE METHODS FOR CLEANING, PACKAGING, STERILIZING, AND DISINFECTING

Rose Seavey, RN, MBA, CNOR, ACSP

As the patient's advocate, the perioperative nurse is responsible for protecting the patient and providing a safe environment for the surgical team. The perioperative nurse and unlicensed team members must make certain that all surgical instruments and medical devices used in procedures are available; are working properly; and have been appropriately cleaned, disinfected, or sterilized according to the Spaulding classification system.

With the Spaulding system, the level of disinfection needed is based on the nature of the item and how it will be used. Devices that are used on sterile tissue are categorized as critical and must be sterile. Devices that come in contact with mucous membranes or nonintact skin are considered semi-critical and must be high-level disinfected immediately before use. Devices that come in contact with intact skin are categorized as noncritical items and should receive intermediate or low-level disinfection.

Case studies, a list of suggested activities, and a bibliographical listing of recommended study materials are provided in this chapter to help you become more proficient in this area of responsibility.

LEARNING OBJECTIVES

Individuals preparing for the CNOR exam will direct their study activities toward obtaining the knowledge and skills required to appropriately and effectively select and use methods for cleaning, packaging, sterilizing, and disinfecting surgical instruments and medical devices.

1. Describe the perioperative nurse's role and responsibilities for selecting and using methods of cleaning, packaging, sterilizing, and disinfecting surgical instruments and medical devices.
2. Discuss the types, uses, and limitation of various sterilization and disinfecting devices.
3. Recognize the role of the perioperative nurse in ensuring surgical instruments and medical devices are adequately disinfected or sterilized.
4. Define the perioperative nurse's responsibilities for maintaining and protecting the integrity of surgical instruments and medical devices.
5. Evaluate the effectiveness of these nursing activities.

TASK STATEMENT; AREAS OF KNOWLEDGE AND SKILL

Task Statement

Apply principles of sterilization, disinfection, cleaning, and packaging and adhere to guidelines set by regulatory agencies and manufacturers to promote safe practice.

Areas of Knowledge

- K-2 Anatomy and physiology
- K-3 Pathophysiology
- K-6 Principles of wound healing
- K-9 Surgical, anesthetic, and other perioperative interventions
- K-11 Physiologic responses to the surgical experience
- K-15 Risks for injury, including but not limited to, skin, positioning, and retained foreign body
- K-17 Postoperative complications
- K-19 Emergency operative procedures
- K-25 *Perioperative Nursing Data Set* (PNDS)
- K-27 Microbiology and infection control
- K-28 Standard and transmission-based precautions

K-31 Technologies and equipment relating to perioperative practice
K-32 Environmental parameters (eg, temperature, humidity, air exchange)
K-33 Principles of sterilization and disinfection
K-34 Protective barrier materials
K-35 Packaging materials
K-36 Principles of equipment inspection, maintenance, and repair
K-37 Principles of product evaluation, cost-containment, and resource management
K-40 Legal responsibilities and implications for patient care
K-43 "ANA Code of Ethics for Nurses with Explications for Perioperative Nurses"
K-44 Regulatory standards and voluntary guidelines
K-45 AORN *Standards, Recommended Practices, and Guidelines*
K-47 Principles of problem solving
K-48 Quality improvement principles
K-53 Rules, responsibilities, and duties of health care team members and internal and external support service personnel
K-56 Implants (eg, handling, tracking, sterilization)

Areas of Skill

S-4 Communicating effectively (verbal and nonverbal)
S-11 Identifying risk of infection and injury
S-15 Collaborating with other members on the health care team
S-16 Applying AORN *Standards, Recommended Practices, and Guidelines*
S-17 Applying the *Perioperative Nursing Data Set* (PNDS)
S-19 Participating in quality improvement activities
S-20 Maintaining accurate patient records
S-21 Protecting patients and members of the health care team from hazardous conditions
S-22 Providing evidence-based care
S-23 Applying regulatory standards and voluntary guidelines
S-25 Apply principles of and participate in cost containment, product evaluation, and resource management
S-27 Delegating interventions and/or assigning tasks
S-28 Adapting to changing situations and technologies
S-29 Performing nursing interventions
S-31 Recording unusual occurrences and/or variances in care
S-36 Applying principles of aseptic technique and infection control
S-37 Applying principles of sterilization and disinfection
S-38 Applying principles of environmental cleaning
S-39 Maintaining a sterile field
S-40 Preparing the surgical site
S-41 Selecting appropriate protective barrier materials
S-42 Conducting biological monitoring
S-44 Testing and using equipment
S-47 Documenting maintenance of a safe environment
S-50 Adapting to special and unusual needs
S-53 Educating, mentoring, and supervising health care team members
S-57 Performing sterilization procedures and conducting monitoring techniques (eg, chemical, biological monitoring and mechanical indicators)
S-58 Identifying appropriate packaging materials for sterilization
S-59 Selecting appropriate and cost-effective sterilization methods

PREOPERATIVE NURSING ACTIVITIES

As part of the surgical team, the perioperative nurse is responsible for providing surgical instruments and medical devices that are safe to use for patient care. To ensure the devices are safe to use on the patient, careful attention to detail and following recommended practices and manufacturers' recommendations are essential.

The perioperative nurse's responsibilities regarding surgical instruments and medical devices during the preoperative period are to ensure that

- the appropriate instruments, supplies, and medical devices, according to the surgeon's preference, are available and safe for use;
- disinfection solutions are at an acceptable level of active ingredient and the temperature of the solution is according to manufacturers' recommendations;
- all sterilizers have had appropriate tests preformed;
- mechanical indicators on the sterilizer equipment are acceptable (eg, right temperature for correct amount of time);
- the integrity of the sterilization packaging is intact and sterility has not been compromised;
- the external chemical indicators have turned the appropriate color, which verifies exposure to the sterilization process; and

- instruments and medical devices are in good condition, function properly, and are complete.

INTRAOPERATIVE NURSING ACTIVITIES

The perioperative nurse must collaborate with all health care workers present in the OR on providing and maintaining a safe environment. Adherence to aseptic practices is a fundamental area of accountability for the perioperative nurse. During the intraoperative period, there are many principals to consider in regard to ensuring instruments and medical devices are safe for patient use.

Surgical instruments and medical devices must be packaged so that their sterility can be maintained until they are opened.

All items should be inspected immediately before use on the sterile field for proper packaging, complete closure, package integrity, and insertion of a sterilization indicator.

There are three basic types of packaging systems used to maintain sterility.

- Wrappers, which can be made of either woven or non-woven material. All wrappers must be inspected for holes, tears, or water spots before being used.
- Peel pouches, which are made out of paper and plastic or paper and Tyvec, depending on the type of sterilization needed. Peel packs are clear on one side, which allows you to view the package contents. Peel packs also must be inspected for holes, tears, or water spots before being used.
- Ridged containers are specially designed metal or plastic cases. These containers help protect surgical instruments. Containers have a filter and/or valve system that allows for the sterilant to enter and protects the contents from contamination after the sterilization cycle. Breakaway locks must be intact to secure the lid and ensure sterility of contents. These locks must be checked to ensure that they are secure and intact before the container is opened.

The packaging system must

- be of appropriate size to protect the contents;
- allow for aseptic presentation;
- be intact with no holes, tears, or water spots;
- be suitable to the method of sterilization according to the manufacturer of the sterilizer or instrument;
- have identification of contents on the outside of the package;
- have a label on the outside with a description of the package contents, initials of the package assembler, and a lot control number;
- have a chemical indicator on the outside that has turned the appropriate color to indicate it has been exposed to the sterilization process; and
- have a favorable cost/benefit ratio.

Surgical instruments should be handled carefully during the surgical procedure to help ensure effectiveness of the instruments and reduce the risk of injury and/or delays.

Instruments should be used only for their intended purpose (eg, tissue scissors should not be used to cut sutures, hemostats should not be used as towel clips, needle drivers should be of appropriate size for the needle used).

Throughout the surgical procedure, instruments should be kept free of gross soil by cleaning the instruments with sterile water and a sponge. Saline, blood, or tissue left on may cause pitting, rusting, staining, or deterioration of the instrument surface. Cannulated or lumened instruments should be irrigated frequently with sterile water to eliminate obstruction.

The nurse may have to sterilize or high-level disinfect surgical instruments immediately before or during the surgical procedure.

Steam Sterilization

Steam sterilization using the unwrapped method is called "flash" sterilization. This method should be considered only if

- the instruments have been properly inspected, cleaned, and decontaminated;
- the sterilizer is located in an area that allows for direct aseptic delivery of the sterilized instruments to the sterile field; and

- aseptic technique is carefully followed when handling and transferring the sterile items.

Sterilizer and instrument manufacturers' written instruction for exposure times and temperature settings should be followed carefully to ensure sterilization is achieved. When sterilizing items needing different exposure times and/or temperature settings (eg, lumened or porous instruments containing rubber or plastic), the most challenging method should be used. For each sterilization cycle, the mechanical parameters of time, temperature, and pressure should be examined, monitored, and recorded to ensure sterility has been achieved. Each sterilizer load must contain a sterilization process monitoring device. Flash sterilizers should be monitored with a biological indicator (BI) daily.

The two most common types of sterilizers used in the OR are gravity displacement or prevacuum. According to the Association for the Advancement of Medical Instrumentation (AAMI), temperature settings for both the gravity displacement and prevacuum sterilizers should be 270-272° F (132-135° C). The exposure time for metal, or nonporous items only in both types of sterilizers is 3 minutes. If items have lumens or porous items (eg, rubber, plastic) the exposure time needed in a gravity cycle is 10 minutes and 4 minutes for a prevacuum cycle.

Instruments with multiple parts must be disassembled before they can be sterilized. Instruments should be placed in a mesh bottom or perforated tray when using the flash method of sterilization. To ensure air removal and steam penetration, solid containers or containers with lids should not be used for this purpose.

Some sterilizers allow for items to be wrapped and flashed, but they must be designed and labeled as such. The sterilizer manufacturer's written recommendations for flashed items must be followed.

Items that will be implanted in the patient should not be flashed sterilized due to possible patient complications. The need to "flash" sterilize implants can be avoided by careful planning, scheduling, and inventory management of the implants. If it is necessary to sterilize an implantable device within the hospital, a biological monitor must be used. AAMI recommends that these implantable devices not be used until the results of a negative biological readout are complete. The flashed implants must be used immediately or reprocessed if needed for a future case.

Peracetic Acid Sterilization

Peracetic acid is a low temperature sterilization process using a liquid chemical solution. This method is used for immersible surgical instruments and/or equipment and is a just-in-time sterilization process. Immersed items cannot be wrapped; therefore, there is no shelf life of items sterilized by this method.

As with flash sterilization, items must be completely cleaned and disassembled before the sterilization process. The manufacturers' written recommendations must be followed for preparation of the instruments or equipment before sterilization. Peracetic acid solution must come in contact with all external and internal surfaces for the specific amount of time. The manufacturers' specifically designed trays and or containers must be used to hold the devices in the correct position. If the surgical instrument or medical device has lumens, fluid flow connectors specifically made for this purpose must be used.

The perioperative nurse or other members of the surgical team must check the printed document after each cycle to make sure that all of the manufacturers recommended parameters are met. The liquid sterilant must reach a temperature of 122-131° F (50-69° C) for a period of 12 minutes. After exposure to the sterilant, the processor will automatically advance through several stages of the rinse cycle. Peracetic acid processing devices have a specific chemical indicator and BI. Each load must contain a chemical indicator that must be checked before the items are used on the patient. It is recommended that these processors be monitored with a BI daily.

High-Level Disinfection

Items that come in contact with nonintact skin or mucous membranes (considered semi-critical devices) should, at the minimum, receive high-level disinfection just before use. There are many high-level disinfection chemical products on the market (eg, glutaraldehyde, peracetic acid, hydrogen peroxide). Some examples of devices that may be high-level disinfection are bronchoscopes, cystoscopes, respiratory therapy equipment, anesthesia equipment, or gastrointestinal endoscopes.

The chemical disinfectant manufacturers' and the device manufacturers' written recommendations must be meticulously followed. Materials compatibility must be checked before use. The devices must be completely submerged for a specific amount of time, depending on the product being used. All chemical disinfectants should be checked before use with an FDA approved product (eg, test strip) to be sure there is a minimal level of concentration of the solution. Some products may have to be heated to a certain temperature to be effective.

Surgical instruments or medical devices must be thoroughly cleaned and disassembled before disinfection procedures. All lumens must be irrigated with the solution while immersed to eliminate any air pockets and make certain there is contact with all internal surfaces. Devices must be thoroughly rinsed with sterile water according to manufacturers' recommendations.

To decrease the possibility of exposure to skin or mucous membranes, personal protective equipment (PPE) should be worn when using liquid chemicals. The PPE may include eyewear and chemical resistant gloves, masks, gown, or other skin protection.

Chemical disinfectant vapors may be toxic; therefore, they should be covered at all times and used in a well-ventilated area. The Occupational Safety and Health Administration (OSHA), which has established exposure limits, regulates occupational exposure to toxic chemicals in the workplace. Facilities are required by law to follow the OSHA limits.

POSTOPERATIVE NURSING ACTIVITIES

When the surgery or invasive procedure is completed, cleaning and decontaminating instruments and equipment should begin at once. All instruments opened and placed on the sterile field may be exposed to splashing of blood, saline, or debris; therefore, they should be considered contaminated and must be decontaminated whether actually used in the procedure or not. Instruments should be dissembled at the point of use and arranged with care in mesh-bottom trays. When preparing instruments for decontamination, the perioperative nurse or unlicensed personnel must

- throw away disposable sharps in an appropriate sharps container,
- put reusable sharp instruments in a separate tray,
- take apart instruments with removable parts,
- open all box locks,
- protect scissors and delicate instruments by placing them on top, and
- separate heavy instruments such as mallets or heavy retractors in a separate tray.

Decontamination

Transportation

The decontamination area may be within the OR or centrally located in the sterile processing/central service department. Instruments should be transported to the decontamination area as soon as possible. Instruments may be covered with a damp towel to prevent drying during transportation. All instruments should be transported in a tightly covered, leak-proof container or may be covered with a plastic bag to minimize potential exposure. Basins filled with water should not be used to transport contaminated instruments due to the potential for spillage.

Personal Protective Equipment (PPE)

Employees working in decontamination must wear surgical scrubs and PPE, which includes hair coverings, an impervious barrier (ie, a gown, jumpsuit, or apron with sleeves), mask, shoe covers, heavy duty gloves, and eye protection (eg, wrap around glasses, face shield) whenever there is a potential for splashing.

Decontamination

Decontamination of instruments is necessary to ensure safe handling by assembling and processing personnel. Instruments must first be cleaned of all gross soil before being decontaminated. Detergents, which are agents that lower surface tension and break down fat, oil, and grease, are used for cleaning. Gross soil should be rinsed off with cool water before using a detergent solution. Hot or warm water could result in coagulation of the protein, making it harder to remove. Always use the manufacturers' instructions for correct dilution, solution temperature, and use. Instruments may be soaked in an enzymatic solution to help with hard-to-clean instruments. A detergent with neutral pH should be used for surgical instruments.

Instruments may be decontaminated manually or automatically. Automatic cleaning is preferred over manual washing whenever possible, but some very delicate instruments or nonimmersible instruments require manual cleaning. Manufacturers' written instructions should be followed to ensure instruments are not harmed during the process. Due to their design, some instruments such as bone reamers may require hand washing as well as automatic decontamination.

Lumened instruments, such as suctions and laparoscopic instruments, must be flushed and brushed with detergent and water or enzymatic solution to ensure that no bioburden remains inside. Brushing must be done with a brush with an adequate diameter and length to reach the entire channel. Ultrasonic irrigators and mechanical cleaners are preferable to manually cleaning.

When manually cleaning instruments, care must be taken to decrease aerosolization, or splashing, of infected materials by completely submersing the device and cleaning under water only.

Automatic/Mechanical Instrument Cleaners

There are several types of mechanical cleaners on the market. The manufacturers' recommendations must be completely followed when using automatic cleaners. Washer-decontaminators or washer sterilizers are two of the most common used for surgical instruments.

Washer decontaminators usually have prerinsing, cleaning, rinsing, final rinsing, and drying cycles. They use rotating sprayer arms at top, bottom, and in-between each shelf of instruments. Some may have other added features to enhance the decontamination process.

Sometimes heat-tolerant surgical instruments are processed through a washer sterilizer. The process consists of several washes and rinses, followed by steam sterilization. If items are not meticulously cleaned before being put into the washer sterilizer, soil may become baked on during the sterilization cycle. Baked-on soil is extremely difficult to clean. If left on it may cause a pyrogen or allergic reaction for the patient.

Ultrasonic Washers

Ultrasonic washers are used to remove fine soil from hard-to-reach places. The ultrasonic machine converts high frequency sound waves into mechanical vibrations, which causes microscopic bubbles to form and implode (ie, burst inward), creating a minute vacuum that draws out debris from the crevices of the instruments. This process is called cavitation. Once instruments are initially cleaned, they may be put into an ultrasonic washer. Due to the aerosolization created by the ultrasonic washer, the cover should be closed when in operation.

Due to the possibility of instrument damage, only instruments of like metal should be put in the ultrasonic cleaner together. Some instruments, such as very delicate instruments, may be damaged in the ultrasonic cleaner. Manufacturers' instructions should be checked before using an ultrasonic cleaner.

Ultrasonic cleaning does not kill microorganisms; it only removes particles that are deposited in the water. Thorough rinsing is necessary after ultrasonic cleaning to remove all of the fine debris. Ultrasonic cleaning should be done in the decontamination area, as opposed to the clean area where items are being assembled, packaged, and sterilized.

Specialty Instruments

Specialty instruments require detailed cleaning and handling. Powered surgical instruments, such as saws and drills or electronic devices, should never be immersed or placed in an ultrasonic cleaner. Permanent damage may result if water enters the internal mechanisms of these devices. As with all specialty instruments, manufacturers' instructions on care and handling should be followed carefully. Powered instruments usually require disassembling and manual cleaning.

Flexible endoscopes are challenging to clean because of their long lumens, valves, and other parts. Instructions are quite specific to the type of scope and must be followed precisely to ensure thorough cleaning and disinfecting. According to AORN's recommended practices, "Personnel should demonstrate competency regarding appropriate selection, proper handling, inspection, testing, use, and processing of endoscopes and related equipment."

Preparation and Sterilization

Instruments should be inspected for cleanliness and defects (eg, cracks, loose screws, nicks, burs) before being assembled into sets or packaging. Sharps must be protected and all box locks should be in an open position. Delicate and lighter instruments should be placed on top of heavier instruments.

Steam Sterilization

Saturated steam under pressure is the most cost-effective and widely used sterilization method for heat and moisture tolerant devices. The effectiveness of steam sterilization depends on direct surface contact of the device and successful vaporization of the water condensate.

There are several types of steam sterilization used in health care facilities. The two most frequently used types are

- gravity displacement, in which steam enters the top of the chamber and pushes the air out the drain at the bottom of the chamber; and

- prevacuum, in which a vacuum system mechanically pulls the air from the sterilizer chamber out drains at the bottom of the chamber.

The most common exposure temperature used is 270° F for a 4-minute cycle. Follow the manufacturer's directions carefully for the type of sterilizer used.

Ethylene Oxide (EO) Sterilization

Ethylene oxide sterilization is used for items that are heat or moisture sensitive and cannot withstand steam sterilization. The EO gas kills microbes under the correct parameters. The essential parameters for sterilization are temperature, exposure time, relative humidity, and concentration of the sterilant. There are several models and manufacturers of EO sterilizers. All items must be aerated (usually 8-12 hours) immediately after exposure to the EO gas to reduce the levels of toxic chemicals. The EO gas is known to be hazardous due to its toxicity; therefore, specific precautions must be observed.

Low Temperature Gas Plasma Sterilization

Low temperature gas plasma sterilization is used for items that are heat or moisture sensitive. Gas plasma does not require an aeration phase. The sterilization cycle is approximately 45-70 minutes. There are some restrictions as to the type of devices that can be sterilized in this system. These sterilizers must be used and monitored according to the manufacturers' written recommendations.

SUMMARY

The perioperative nurse should be aware of the recommendations that provide guidance for the use and methods of sterilization, disinfection, and packaging of surgical instruments and medical devices. Manufacturers' written recommendations of the device and the equipment must be followed to ensure safe patient care.

CASE STUDIES

Case Study: Scenario A

You are the circulator preparing the OR for a laparoscopic cholecystectomy. When opening the ridged container of laparoscopic instruments, you notice that the filter in the top of the sterilization container is intact. When the scrub person removes the basket of instruments, you notice the filter is missing from the bottom of the container. The scrub person has already placed the instrument container on the sterile back table.

Points to Consider

- Are these instruments safe for patient use?
- Is the back table and its contents contaminated?
- Is the scrub person contaminated?
- What steps need to be taken before the procedure can begin?
- Are there other instruments that can be substituted?
- What can be done to eliminate this in the future?

Discussion of Points to Consider

Your responses should have included the following points:

- What are the manufacturer's recommended guidelines for the use of ridged container systems? Some containers have solid bottoms and a filter only on the top. Are there perforations on the bottom of the container where the filters are suppose to be?
- Filters are necessary to allow air removal and entry of the sterilant. If the filter is missing, the instruments must be considered unsterile and not be used.
- The back table and the scrub person must be considered contaminated. The scrub person must regown and reglove, and the back table cover must be removed and redrapped.
- The laparoscopic instruments are considered not sterile, and other instruments must be used. If there are not other like pans of instruments, and the instruments are steam tolerant, they may be flashed sterilized.
- It is imperative that the filters and or valve assembly on instrument containers be checked for completeness and inspected for holes before items are placed on the sterile field. In addition, the perioperative nurse should check to see if the chemical indicators have changed color and that the locks are intact before use.

Case Study: Scenario B

You are the scrub person on an open orthopedic case. The procedure requires the use of a power drill. When setting up the case, you notice that the detachable hand piece is already attached to the air hose.

Points to Consider

- Should you use this drill on this surgical procedure?
- What are the manufacturer's recommendation for cleaning and sterilizing?
- Has this handpiece been removed for cleaning, or did it go though the cleaning and sterilizing process while still together?
- Is there another drill that can be used?
- How can we help prevent this in the future?

Discussion of Points to Consider

- Powered surgical instruments usually require disassembling and manual cleaning.
- The drill should be considered contaminated. Sterilization is dependant on reaching all surfaces, and when an item is not disassembled for cleaning and sterilization, sterility cannot be ensured.
- Because you are not sure if this drill has been cleaned properly, it must be cleaned properly before it can be resterilized.
- Another drill must be used for the case.
- To help prevent this in the future, it is important to follow up with the person who assembled and wrapped the drill prior to sterilization. The initials of the person should be on the container.
- It also is important to remind all scrub personnel to disassemble the hand piece from the power cord before sending the instruments to the decontamination area. Protecting the patient and the instruments is the responsibility of the entire surgical team, which includes sterile processing/central service staff members.

SUGGESTED LEARNING ACTIVITIES

◆ Review the current AORN Recommended Practices for: High-Level Disinfection; Use and Care of Endoscopes; Cleaning and Caring for Surgical Instruments and Powered Equipment; Selection and Use of Packaging Systems; Maintaining a Sterile Field; Sterilization in Perioperative Practice Settings. If you have any questions or comments, contact the AORN staff in the Center for Nursing Practice.

◆ Review the safety requirements for handling contaminated items and body fluids, toxic chemical used for disinfection and sterilization from AORN, AAMI, and OSHA.

◆ Become familiar with the manufacturers' written recommendations for all equipment and instruments.

◆ Spend time in the sterile processing/central service department to understand the process in your facility for cleaning, packaging, sterilization, and disinfection.

◆ Keep current in these subject areas by reviewing the literature in perioperative nursing and infection control journals.

RECOMMENDED STUDY MATERIALS

AAMI, *Standards and Recommended Practices. Sterilization, Parts 1, 2, 3: Sterilization in Health Care Facilities* Vols 1.1, 1.2, 1.3 (Arlington, Va: American Association for Medical Instrumentation, 2001).

AORN, *Standards, Recommended Practices, and Guidelines* (Denver: AORN, Inc, 2002).

ASHCSP, *Recommended Practice for Central Service,* "Section Four: Assembly and Packaging" (Chicago: American Society for Healthcare Central Service Professionals of the American Hospital Association, 1999).

ASHCSP, *Recommended Practice for Central Service,* "Section Three: Decontamination," (Chicago: American Society for Healthcare Central Service Professionals of the American Hospital Association, 1999).

ASHCSP, *Recommended Practice for Central Service,* "Section Six: Sterilization," (Chicago: American Society for Healthcare Central Service Professionals of the American Hospital Association, 1999).

ASHCSP, *Training Manual for Central Service Technicians*, fourth ed (Chicago: American Society for Healthcare Central Service Professionals of the American Hospital Association, 2001).

Brooks Tighe, S, *Instrumentation for the Operation Room: A Photographic Manual* fifth ed (St Louis: Mosby, Inc, 1999).

CHAPTER 15: EMERGENCY SITUATIONS

Linda Brazen, RN, MSN, CNOR

A perioperative nurse's response to emergency patient situations, regardless of the nature of the situation, is very similar to his or her response during any and all patient care activities, with the exception of time. The accountability and responsibility of a perioperative nurse, regardless of the situation, should be focused on two core patient outcomes—keeping the patient free from injury and keeping the patient free from infection. During the usual day-to-day activities, basic patient care needs are assessed and identified in relation to the outcomes, individualized complementary care activities are planned and implemented, and patient needs in relation to the nursing activities and outcomes are evaluated. During an emergency patient situation, the accountability, responsibility, outcomes, patient needs, care activities, and evaluation are performed as seemingly one response.

This chapter describes the variety and diversity of emergency patient situations that perioperative nurses may encounter in their practice. The knowledge and skill required in these situations vary depending on the role(s) that the perioperative nurse may assume during emergency responses. The roles vary depending on the emergent nature of the situation (eg, internal, external, preoperative, intraoperative, postoperative) or based on a patient need. It is important to note, however, that as the requirement for perioperative nurses preparing for certification is based on experience, and the experience depends on basic and continuing medical-surgical knowledge, it is not within the purpose of this chapter to present foundations of pathophysiology or pathology. The importance of the perioperative nurse's ability in an emergency patient situation relies on three abilities that all must function simultaneously while assessing changing patient care needs. These abilities are to

- subjectively prioritize; think critically; react responsively; and at times delegate and/or assume supportive, assistive, and reactive roles;
- perform only within the scope of his or her practice as a nurse; and
- direct, coordinate, and manage the nursing care needs of patients through manipulating others such as peers and unlicensed staff (ie, delegation), supplies, equipment, and ongoing objective and subjective data from assessment and reassessment sources.

LEARNING OBJECTIVES

1. Describe the causes and complications of common perioperative patient emergency situations.
2. Describe the causes and complications of common perioperative internal emergency situations.
3. Describe the causes and complications of common perioperative external emergency situations.
4. Describe role(s) perioperative nurses may assume during any type of perioperative emergency situation.
5. Discuss the requisite abilities of a perioperative nurse while he or she is continuously assessing changing patient care needs in response to an emergency situation.

TASK STATEMENT; AREAS OF KNOWLEDGE AND SKILL

Task Statement

Plan for and implement nursing activities to provide care in an emergency situation.

Areas of Knowledge

K-1 Health assessment techniques
K-2 Anatomy and physiology
K-3 Pathophysiology
K-4 Pharmacology and anesthetic agents
K-5 Pain management
K-7 Diagnostic procedures and results
K-8 Preoperative patient preparation activities
K-9 Surgical, anesthetic, and other perioperative interventions
K-10 Expected outcomes related to identified interventions
K-11 Physiologic responses to the surgical experience
K-12 Principles of positioning
K-13 Ergonomics and body mechanics
K-14 Transfer and transport techniques and equipment
K-15 Risks for injury, including, but not limited to, skin, positioning and retained foreign body
K-16 Emergency procedures (eg, CPR, MH)
K-17 Postoperative complications
K-18 Defining characteristics of impending patient physiologic crisis
K-19 Emergency operative procedures
K-20 Sociology (eg, cultural and ethnic influences, family patterns, spirituality and related practices)
K-21 Communication theories and techniques
K-22 Behavioral responses to the surgical experience
K-23 Discharge planning
K-25 *Perioperative Nursing Data Set* (PNDS)
K-26 Requirements for handling of specimens
K-27 Microbiology and infection control
K-28 Standard and transmission-based precautions
K-29 Potential hazards in the perioperative environment, including, but not limited to, chemical, electrical, fire, gas, laser, physical environment, radiologic, extraneous objects
K-30 Interventions to optimize safety
K-31 Technologies and equipment relating to perioperative practice
K-32 Environmental parameters (eg, temperature, humidity, air exchange)
K-33 Principles of sterilization and disinfection
K-34 Protective barrier materials
K-37 Principles of product evaluation, cost containment, and resource management
K-38 Emergency preparedness (eg, fire, disaster)
K-39 Patient rights and responsibilities
K-40 Legal responsibilities and implications for patient care
K-41 Approved nursing diagnoses (eg, NANDA)
K-42 Nursing research and evidence-based practice
K-43 "ANA Code of Ethics for Nurses with Explications for Perioperative Nurses"
K-44 Regulatory standards and voluntary guidelines
K-45 AORN *Standards, Recommended Practices, and Guidelines*
K-46 AORN position statements (eg, bloodborne pathogens, do-not-resuscitate orders [DNR])
K-47 Principles of problem solving
K-49 Surgical consent laws and policies
K-50 Defining characteristics of impaired individuals (eg, substance abuse, psychological disturbance, compromised performance)
K-52 Defining characteristics of domestic abuse (eg, child, elder, partner/spouse)
K-53 Rules, responsibilities, and duties of health care team members, and internal and external support service personnel
K-54 Organ procurement
K-55 Credentialing standards and clinical privileges
K-56 Implants (handling, tracking, sterilization)

Areas of Skill

S-1 Confirming patient identity, operative site, and procedure
S-2 Collecting, analyzing, and prioritizing patient data
S-3 Using health assessment techniques (eg, interview, observation, auscultation, palpation, percussion)
S-4 Communicating effectively (verbal and nonverbal)
S-5 Advocating and protecting patient rights
S-7 Assessing and managing pain
S-8 Assessing for potential abuse (eg, substance, domestic)
S-11 Identifying risk of infection and injury
S-12 Identifying cultural, spiritual, ethnic issues in care
S-13 Identifying age specific needs
S-15 Collaborating with other members on the health care team
S-16 Applying AORN *Standards, Recommended Practices, and Guidelines*
S-17 Applying the *Perioperative Nursing Data Set* (PNDS)
S-10 Participating in quality improvement activities
S-20 Maintaining accurate patient records
S-21 Protecting patients and members of the health care team from hazardous conditions
S-22 Providing evidence based care
S-23 Applying regulatory standards and voluntary guidelines
S-27 Delegating interventions and/or assigning tasks
S-28 Adapting to changing situations and technologies
S-29 Performing nursing interventions

S-30 Documenting all relevant facts and data elements with appropriate terminology
S-31 Recording unusual occurrences and/or variances in care
S-32 Applying principles and techniques of transport, transfer, and positioning
S-33 Anticipating the needs for equipment, supplies, and personnel
S-34 Applying principles and techniques of body mechanics/ergonomics
S-35 Maintaining the dignity, modesty, and privacy of the patient and protecting the confidentiality of patient information
S-36 Applying principles of aseptic technique and infection control
S-39 Maintaining a sterile field
S-40 Preparing the surgical site
S-44 Testing and using equipment
S-46 Anticipating and evaluating the effects of pharmacological and anesthetic agents
S-48 Detecting significant changes in the environment
S-50 Adapting to special and unusual needs
S-51 Identifying and communicating changes in patient status
S-52 Documenting nursing interventions and patient response
S-53 Educating, mentoring, and supervising health care team members
S-54 Recognizing impaired behavior in patients, family, and staff and responding appropriately
S-55 Recognizing personal limitations and seeking assistance as needed
S-56 Measuring, evaluating, and documenting patient outcomes
S-60 Directing health care team members in emergency situations
S-61 Performing basic life support and other emergency procedures
S-62 Setting priorities
S-65 Applying ethical principles
S-67 Evaluating for signs and symptoms of injury
S-69 Recording devices implanted or explanted during procedures

OVERVIEW

The patient's medical history and physical and perioperative nursing assessment should include a review of systems, prescribed medications and self-prescribed therapies, and baseline data regarding respiratory, circulatory, skin integrity, mobility and pain scale, as well as level of consciousness. The patient's readiness to learn and supportive information are assessed, and all is considered in developing an individualized plan of care and managing and coordinating that care through the perioperative continuum. Patients who do not appear to be compromised, patients assessed to be minimally compromised, and those who are extremely compromised in any assessment data share an equal potential to be in need of emergency response.

As a perioperative nurse collects baseline data during the patient's preoperative interview, he or she must be able to manipulate the data to identify compromises a patient presents and plan and implement care activities that decrease the patient's potential of needing an emergency response. Alternately, patients may present in various states of need such that they are unable to participate in a preoperative interview, already having experienced an emergency response in the field, or about who minimal known data is available or known (eg, John Doe). In lieu of an intensive assessment phase, the perioperative RN must use emergency response knowledge and skill to pre-plan nursing care activities that decrease the patient's potential for an(other) emergency response. If time is extremely limited, the RN may need to rely on the field assessment performed under the mnemonic "AMPLE":

- A—assessment of allergies,
- M—medications/recreational drug use,
- P—past medical/operative history,
- L—last meal/last tetanus, and
- E—events leading to the injury.[1]

Table 1 lists the more common types of compromises a patient may present with and/or may have potential to manifest during operative procedures. The patient data to be assessed for each of these compromises may be objective or subjective. The compromise itself may precipitate an emergency response or many compromises may potentiate an emergency response. Some of the compromises themselves are of major significance whereas some are significant only if they are a concurrent compromise. The list is a basic reference, not a sole source for patients in need of emergency responses.

The Role of the Perioperative Nurse

The role of the perioperative nurse in patient-centered emergency responses remains the same as if the patient is under usual-and-customary perioperative care. He or she advocates for the patient, and is supportive, reactive, and responsive to changing patient needs and continuous and multiple requests. The nurse also will need to manage and coordinate nursing care activities that promote freedom from infection and freedom from injury for the patient. Prioritizing demands, while performing activities in their order of priority, and the ability to delegate to others based on their qualifications and competence are requisite skills. Table 2 lists emergency response nursing diagnoses related to common patient compromises.

COMMON PATIENT EMERGENCY SITUATIONS

Patient-centered situations that potentiate emergency responses may present as a pathology of the patient, and why the patient is in need of an operative procedure. These situations may be observable, may be identified in the patient's medical history or physical, or may be a situation that is discovered during a caregiver's assessment interview. Pathological causes potentiate most compromise to the ABC systems: A—airway, B—breathing, and C—circulation.

- *Example*—A patient presents with an observable pathology of a goiter; alternately the patient may present with a written diagnosis of carcinoma of the larynx which, through a review of the medical history, the perioperative RN discovers is a tumor that is sized and located such that it will potentially obstruct the patient's airway when the anesthesia care provider performs a jaw thrust for intubation.
    - The *patient outcome* focus during the *nursing assessment* activity in both of these patient-centered situations is to keep the patient free from injury.
    - The *planning and implementation* of nursing activities in both patient-centered situations is to access the airway management supplies and equipment as part of the scheduled case.
    - The *role of the nurse* in both patient-centered situation is assistive, as necessary. He or she also manages, coordinates, and delegates appropriate activities if emergency responses are necessary.

A second line of patient-centered situations that potentiate emergency responses may result from a patient's systems deficit, or if one of their systems compensates for another system. It may be that these system(s) deficits also are related to their need for an operative procedure, but manifest in a preoperative, intraoperative, and/or postoperative phase of care. The basic human systems, (ie, integumentary, musculoskeletal, neurological, circulatory, respiratory, genitourinary, gastro-intestinal) need to be considered as needs for potential emergency responses.

- *Example*—Patients with chronic conditions in systems also usually are on various medications that increase the potential for emergency response (eg, beta-blockers).

- *Example*—Patients with chronic conditions may compromise a system by their use of over-the-counter (OTC) therapies, herbal remedies, and

TABLE 1
Common Patient-Centered Compromises of Significance to Perioperative Nurses

Preoperative
- chest pain
- penetrating trauma
- procedural pain (IV catheter, anesthetic block)
- anesthesia risk factors
- history of untoward reaction to anesthetic agents
- history of chronic conditions/treatment/medication
- status of dentition
- NPO status

Intraoperative
- air embolism
- pulmonary embolism
- arrythmia
- malignant hyperthermia syndrome
- positioning
- difficult intubation
- temperature regulation
- hypoxemia and hypercapnia during anesthesia
- physiologic disturbances due to induced condition during operative and other invasive procedure (eg, hypothermic cardiac bypass)
- bronchospasm

Postoperative
- hemorrhagic shock
- hypoxemia/hypercapnia postanesthesia
- anesthesia-related trauma caused by surgical malpositioning
- postoperative emotional response
- nausea or vomiting
- allergic reactions

alternate therapies.

- The *patient outcome* focus during the *nursing assessment* is to keep the patient free from injury.
- The *planning and implementation* of nursing activities is to consider alternate systems that may be compromised.
    - o Beta-blockers block sympathetic responses.
    - o Licorice increases the potential for hypertensive episodes.
    - o Simple common aspirin increases the potential for coagulopathies.
- The *role of the nurse* in this type of patient-centered situation is to manage the patient's care by ensuring emergency response supplies (including blood products) and equipment are available and in working order, and ensuring their own competence to use the equipment is current.

Another line of patient-centered situations that potentiate emergency responses may result from a care provider's approach (or lack thereof) to managing a patient's system(s) while the patient is undergoing the operative procedure. The management of airway, fluids, the operative site as well as preoperative and postoperative pain management, and managing the patient's need for information/education are within this line of patient-centered situations that may potentiate an emergency response.

◆ *Example*—Patients with poor skin integrity, specifically neonates and the elderly.
- The *patient outcome* focus during the nursing assessment is to keep the patient free from injury.
- The *planning and implementation* of nursing activities is toward supporting skin integrity because poor skin integrity increases the potential for neurological system compromise and circulatory system compromise which, in turn, potentiate pressure, rub, and friction from the bed linen

TABLE 2
Emergency Response Nursing Diagnoses Related to Common Patient Compromises

Nursing Diagnosis	Patient Compromise
Ineffective airway/ impaired gas exchange	Head/neck trauma Altered level of consciousness Aspiration/aspiration pneumonia Effects of anesthetic, operative procedure, surgical positioning
Fluid volume deficit	Nature of injury Overt hemmorhage Resuscitative fluid and medication treatment(s) pre-admission
Situational anxiety	Related to unexpected trauma Unfamiliar environment (hospital, OR) Concern for others significant to the patient Impending operative/invasive procedures Related to pain Related to body image
Impaired tissue integrity	Related to nature of injury Related to surgical positioning Related to pre-existing medical conditions Related to length of operative procedure
Ineffective thermoregulation	Related to resuscitative fluid management Related to nature of injury Related to surgical exposure Related to shock

and emergency responses.

- The *role of the nurse* is to ensure patients with age-specific special needs that potentiate multiple-systems challenges are appropriately positioned and padded for the procedure.

COMMON EMERGENCY SITUATIONS: INTERNAL

Management of the patient's preoperative, intraoperative, and postoperative care environment and managing the entire perioperative environment is another responsibility of a perioperative nurse. This includes, but is not limited to, situations such as latex sensitivities, ambient temperature, electrotrauma, fire, and explosions. The accountability and responsibility of a perioperative nurse continues to focus on the same two patient outcomes—freedom from injury and freedom from infection. The two outcomes can be used to categorize types of situations in the internal environment that precipitate the need for an emergency response and/or may potentiate the need for an emergency response. The two outcomes can be referenced

Table 3
Emergent Response Practices Related to Compromised Outcomes

AORN Recommended Practice	Patient Outcome
Anesthesia equipment—cleaning and processing	Freedom from infection Freedom from injury
Attire, surgical	Freedom from injury
Conscious sedation/analgesia—Managing the patient	Freedom from injury
Counts-Sponge, sharp, and instrument	Freedom from injury Freedom from infection
Disinfection, high-level	Freedom from injury Freedom from infection
Electrosurgery	Freedom from injury
Environmental cleaning in the surgical practice setting	Freedom from infection Freedom from injury
Hand scrubs, surgical	Freedom from infection
Hazards in the surgical environment	Freedom from injury
Instruments and powered equipment—Care and cleaning	Freedom from infection Freedom from injury
Laser safety in practice settings	Freedom from injury
Local anesthesia—Managing the patient	Freedom from injury
Pneumatic tourniquet	Freedom from injury
Positioning the patient in the perioperative practice setting	Freedom from injury
Reducing radiological exposure in the practice setting	Freedom from injury
Skin preparation of patients	Freedom from infection Freedom from injury
Standard and transmission-based precautions	Freedom from infection
Sterile field—Maintaining	Freedom from infection
Sterilization in the practice setting	Freedom from infection
Traffic patterns in the perioperative setting	Freedom from infection

within certain AORN recommended practices as a conceptual guide for managing the patient's environment and thc perioperative environment. Table 3 lists AORN recommended practices related to patient outcomes; compromise to practice in turn compromise outcome(s) and in turn create the potential for emergency response situations.

- *Example*—"Recommended practices for safe care through identification of potential hazards in the surgical environment"
  - The *patient outcome* focus during the nursing assessment of the patient's environment (ie, OR) and/or the nursing assessment of the overall perioperative environment is the same—freedom from injury.
  - The *planning and implementation* of nursing activities is two-fold in the event the patient is in need of an emergency response.
    - o The OR environment proper is free of extraneous supplies and equipment so that an emergency response, if necessary, can occur without
      - injury to the patient due to inaccessibility to provide emergency care,
      - injury to the responders due to extension cords, low clearance, slippage, body mechanics (eg, lifting), or
      - injury to the responders due to excessive supplies, equipment, furniture in hallways/corridors, emergency response carts inappropriately placed or in a place that is inaccessible due to supplies, equipment, or furniture that has not been returned to its proper place and by nature of inaccessibility does not allow timely assistance.
  - The *role of the nurse* is to establish both safe OR environments and safe perioperative environments, to continuously manage and monitor both environments, and coordinate and delegate appropriate activities if emergency responses are necessary.

- *Example*—"Recommended practices for maintaining a sterile field"
  - The *patient outcome* focus during the nursing assessment of the sterile field is freedom from infection.
  - The *planning and implementation* of nursing activities in the case of an untoward event, emergency response, or compromise to the integrity of the field may include, but are not limited to, advocating for the patient's outcome:
    - o identification of breaks in aseptic technique,
    - o providing supplies, equipment, and direction for corrective actions (eg, removing a contaminated glove), and
    - o using standard precautions based practices.
  - The *role of the nurse* is to establish both a safe OR environment and a safe perioperative environment. Once established, the perioperative nurse monitors/manages both ambient temperature and humidity, monitors/manages traffic patterns and personnel movement in both environments, and coordinates emergency response supplies and equipment within the sterile field, within the OR, and within the overall perioperative environment.

- *Example*—"Recommended practices for environmental cleaning in the surgical practice setting"
  - The *patient outcome* focus during the nursing assessment of environmental cleaning is both freedom from injury and freedom from infection.
  - The *planning and implementation* of nursing activities simultaneously focus on both outcomes within the perioperative care of the patient and within the care of the patient's care environment and within the perioperative care environment.
    - o For example, if the environmental service providers have not been properly trained in the preparation of disinfectant solutions, residual chemical may remain on the OR bed mattress. The potential for a patient's thermoregulation combined with the ambient temperature and one-time use surgical drapes to create perspiration, or for residual surgical skin preparation solutions to create a "wet" surface on the OR linen, may enhance the residual chemical and result in the patient's potential for a thermal burn or a chemical burn or electric burn.
      - Potential for postoperative infection secondary to intraoperative injury

  - Additionally, the residual chemical on the OR bed mattress in combination with the use of electrosurgical devices potentiates conditions for intraoperative fires.
    - Potential for intraoperative injury secondary to caregiver services
- The *role of the nurse* is to establish safe OR environments and safe perioperative environments through education, training, and supervision of support services. A perioperative nurse is responsible for monitoring/managing both environments for temperature/humidity, the traffic patterns/personnel movements, and if/as needed, coordinates emergency response supplies and equipment within the sterile field, the OR environment and within the overall perioperative environment.

COMMON EMERGENCY SITUATIONS: EXTERNAL

A disaster can be defined by category (ie, major or minor) and by type (ie, internal or external).[2] Internal disasters occur within the facility and are commonly related to "system failures" that disrupt or prevent the delivery of care to patients.[3] External disasters occur outside the facility and range from weather-related natural disasters, community disasters such as structural collapses or school-incidents, or those that can be deliberately created (eg, terrorist attacks).

In external disaster situations, the emergency department is likely to receive a first alert; in turn, the facility safety officer will determine the extent of the disaster, the impact it will have on the facility's resources, priority mobilization of people and equipment, and time it will take to mobilize. Implications for the OR department include canceling elective cases and, perhaps, activating a voluntary call-in of staff who were not scheduled to work. Another option may be to recruit day surgery staff willing and able to supplement the OR staff in an assistive capacity for the duration of the disaster.

Note that all staff members are assigned according to patient needs and their level of competence to deal with potential emergency patient response. In lieu of being competent to provide independent patient care, staff members may assume roles such as staging donated supplies from other facilities/organizations, monitoring for identification badges during security lockdowns, manning the telephones, and creating quiet private places for families or patients' significant others. It is imperative that no patient information gets to the media or others before the family/significant others have been contacted. It also is imperative that perioperative nurses recognize what patient information is within their scope of practice to share versus what information should come from the medical staff (eg, anesthesiologist, surgeon).

Preparing staff for external disaster is an accreditation requirement that includes the need for a department specific disaster plan, an evacuation plan, a semi-annual drill for staff competence in evacuation and/or mass casualty, and a debriefing of the drill. In the case of a real alert, it is recommended that incidental stress debriefing occur on an "as needed" basis. The perioperative nurse may be involved in assessing the need for a debriefing and contacting any number of other resources (eg, human resource staff, mental health staff, social workers).[4]

◆ *Example*—The emergency department is alerted that a local high school has experienced a pepper spray incident during a school assembly. The department anticipates two dozen victims in need of eye irrigations and eye exams. The OR is alerted to the potential need for emergency operative ophthalmic procedures, secondary to irrigations and exams.
  - The *patient outcome* focus during the nursing assessment of external disaster plan is both freedom from injury and freedom from infection.
  - The *planning and implementation* of nursing activities focus on staff in relation to competence and unknown volume of patients with unknown acuities. Pre-planning is a priority that should use the unknowns in relation to the knowns.
    - It may be assumed that most of the victims will be minors.
    - It may be assumed that as the incident occurred during a school day, those who will be in a position of authority need to be contacted and will meet most of the victims in the emergency department triage area.
    - It may be assumed that informed consent may be a challenge.
    - It may be assumed that some form of identification system be established to match victims with adults authorized to consent for them.

- The *role of the nurse* includes, but is not limited to, assessing the availability of OR space and the abilities of staff on duty, assigning personnel and/or providing relief to certain staff to continue care in operating rooms and prepare for incoming victims, assessing ophthalmic supplies and equipment and, as necessary, initiating the borrow system from other facilities.

SUMMARY

Operative risk is the probability of adverse outcome and/or death that is associated with surgery and anesthesia. All patients in need of an operative or other invasive procedure are at operative risk, and some situations place patients in need of emergency response and emergency management during invasive procedures. This chapter identifies three situations that have the potential to place the patient in a "higher" operative risk category (ie, situations that are patient-centered, internal disaster situations, and external disaster situations).

The foci are presented in the context of nursing assessment, patient outcomes, planning, and implementations, and the role of the nurse. Of these, emphasis should be placed on the role of the nurse. Many times, because of experience and/or a relationship with a surgeon or anesthesiologist, a perioperative nurse may instinctively "know" how to "do" a medical activity (eg, place a retractor, place a suture, perform an intravenous catheterization). However, if the activity is (1) not within the scope of nursing or (2) not within the nurse's job description, he or she is practicing medicine without a license and is subject to liability.

Readers preparing for the CNOR exam are encouraged to study skill and knowledge specific to the scope of nursing and, when sitting for the exam, use *nursing* as the guide in selecting the most appropriate response to the items. For example, if a patient is in need of an emergency response secondary to an anesthetic-related risk (eg, malignant hyperthermia), the perioperative nurse's activities are focused on activating the department's emergency response; delegating and directing traffic to secure the sterile field; and simultaneously securing the supplies, equipment, and medication necessary to counteract the manifesting signs and symptoms. To not support the nursing needs of the patient in lieu of starting an arterial line (perhaps *not* within a job description or scope of practice) is to do harm to the patient.

CASE STUDIES

Case Study: Mr. W

Mr. W, a retired chief financial officer of a local manufacturing firm, is brought to the OR for insertion of a permanent pacemaker under local anesthesia. The patient is 67 years old and married with four grown children. His diagnosis is third-degree heart block.

Mr. W is transferred to the OR bed and placed in the supine position. He is prepped and draped in the surgeon's routine manner. The surgeon administers the local anesthetic. During the insertion of the cardiac lead, Mr. W experiences a prolonged episode of premature ventricular contractions (PVCs).

Points to Consider

- In planning for this procedure, what additional equipment would be required?
- In preparing the patient for this procedure, what preoperative preparations would be essential for emergency preparedness?
- In monitoring the patient receiving local anesthesia, what would be your nursing responsibilities?
- As the circulating nurse, what should be your initial response to the episode of PVCs?
- What mediation, dose, and route is the surgeon likely to order in treating the episode of PVCs?

Discussion of Points to Consider

Your responses should have included the following points.

- Additional equipment required:
  - o Emergency drug and supply cart
  - o Defibrillator and ECG monitor
  - o Radiolucent operating bed
  - o Fluoroscopy unit
  - o Lead aprons and shields for patient and staff members
- Preoperative preparations for emergency preparedness:
  - o Insertion of an IV catheter with slow-drip IV solution for emergency venous access, as ordered
  - o Proper placement of ECG electrodes and ensure function of the ECG monitor
  - o Preparation for administration of oxygen per nasal cannula
- Nursing responsibilities in monitoring the patient receiving local anesthesia:

- o Knowledge of the function and use of monitoring equipment and ability to interpret the data obtained
- o Monitoring the reaction to drugs related to physiological and behavioral changes, including blood pressure, heart rate and rhythm, respiratory rate, oxygen saturation, skin condition, mental status
- o Documentation of the patient care provided, which should reflect evidence of continued assessment, planning, implementation, and evaluation

- Circulator's initial response to the episode of PVCs:
  - o Count each occurrence aloud to communicate with the surgeon (without alarming Mr. W), as in "One, one, one, one, one . . ."
- Medication for treatment of PVCs:
  - o Administer lidocaine bolus of 1 mg/kg IV and start lidocaine 2 mg drip upon physician's order or OR protocol

Case Study: Ms. B

Ms. B, who is 26 years old, was driver of a car that was struck on the driver's side by a truck. The patient was wearing a seat belt. She was taken to the emergency room by emergency medical personnel at 11:35 PM. Ms. B presents with left-side injuries. Her left arm and leg are splinted, a cervical collar is in place, and she is on a backboard. The patient is responsive but has no recall of the accident.

Findings upon examination of the patient in the emergency department include:

- Blood in left ear canal and ecchymosis of left mastoid area
- Crepitus and decreased breath sounds, left lung field
- Compressed, comminuted fracture, left humerus
- Left-sided paresthesia
- Possible fractured pelvis, with questionable intra-abdominal injuries
- Fractured left tibia-fibula
- Vital signs: blood pressure = 80/60 (palpated); heart rate = 120/min; respirations = 36/min and labored

The trauma surgeon decides that exploratory surgery is required.

Points to Consider

- With the information you have received, what do you assess as the priority life supporting procedures for Ms. B for which you must make plans?
- What clues would indicate the nursing diagnosis, "Airway clearance, ineffective"?
- What diagnostic reports would be helpful in planning Ms. B's intraoperative care?
- Why would well thought-out and coordinated transfer and positioning procedures be vitally important in obtaining quality patient care outcomes for Ms. B?
- What other procedures may be required preoperatively for Ms. B?
- Upon arrival in the OR, what essential information must you obtain from support service?

Discussion of Points to Consider

Your responses should have included the following points.

- Priority life-supporting procedures for Ms. B:
  - o Airway maintenance
  - o Possible insertion of chest tube in order to treat flail chest
- Clues indicating the nursing diagnosis, "Airway clearance, ineffective":
  - o Crepitus and decreased breath sounds, left lung field
  - o Rapid, labored respirations
- Diagnostic reports that would be helpful in planning Ms. B's intraoperative care:
  - o Arterial blood gases
  - o CT scan of abdomen or peritoneal tap for diagnosis of ruptured viscera, fractured pelvis
  - o CBC especially hemoglobin/hematocrit
  - o Chest x-ray
- Importance of coordinated transfer and positioning procedures to obtain quality patient care outcomes for Ms. B.
  - o Blood in left ear canal, ecchymosis of left mastoid, and left-sided paresthesia may be indicative of basilar skull fracture or cervical fracture. Care will need to be taken to support the head and neck and to move the body as a unit, as well as to maintain proper alignment while supporting fractures of the left extremities, chest, and pelvis to prevent further injury. Directing the health care team in transfer and positioning would ensure that everyone understands his or her role.
- Other procedures that may be required preoperatively for Ms. B:
  - o Insertion of arterial line for invasive monitoring and to obtain ABG samples

  - o Insertion of straight or indwelling urinary catheter (Care would need to be taken to not force the catheter against any resistance, due to possible fractured pelvis and ruptured bladder.)
- Essential information that must be obtained from support service personnel:
  - o Blood availability from blood bank (Potential internal injury clues: dropping blood pressure and rapid heart rate may indicate hemorrhage from ruptured viscera, following blunt trauma from seat belt during accident.)

SUGGESTED LEARNING ACTIVITIES

- ◆ Maintain basic life support knowledge.
- ◆ Review AORN patient outcome standards and recommended practices.
- ◆ Review "AORN Malignant Hyperthermia Guideline" and "AORN Latex Allergy Guideline."
- ◆ Review the table of contents of a current text on anesthesia management; reflect on practice; discuss issues and questions with an anesthesia care provider—remember to focus on nursing knowledge, skill, and ability.
- ◆ Research the literature for perioperative disaster articles; review and reflect on nursing activities in relation to patient care needs.

RECOMMENDED STUDY MATERIALS

Andrews, C, "Preventing air embolism," *American Journal of Nursing* 102 (1) (2002) 34-36.

Breedy, L, et al, *Decision Making in Anesthesiology: An Algorithmic Approach* (St Louis: Mosby, Inc, 2000).

Brown, M; Brown, E, *Comprehensive Postanesthesia Care* (Baltimore: William and Wilkins, 1997).

Burke, M, "Disaster planning in the perioperative environment," in *Perioperative Services,* C Frye, C Spry, eds (Gaithersburg, Md: Aspen Publishers, 2002).

Caldwell, J; Ziglar, M, "Hemmorrhagic shock in children," *American Journal of Nursing* (Sept 2001 supplement) 25-27.

Emde, K; Rush, C, "Suspecting pulmonary embolism," *American Journal of Nursing* (Sept 2001 supplement) 19-24.

Jones, C; Cadwell, "Beat the clock," *American Journal of Nursing* (Sept 2001 supplement) 11-14.

King, C, "Trauma Care," in *Patient Care During Operative and Invasive Procedures,* M L Phippen, M P Wells, eds (Philadelphia: W B Saunders Co, 2000).

Murray, T; Patterson, L, "Prone positioning of trauma patients with acute respiratory distress syndrome and open abdominal incisions," *Critical Care Nurse* 22 (3) (2002) 52-56.

Reeder, R; Danis, D, "Penetrating chest trauma," *American Journal of Nursing* (Sept 2001 supplement) 15-18.

Summer, G; Puntillo, K, "Management of surgical and procedural pain in a critical care setting," *Critical Care Nursing Clinics of North America* 13 (2) (2001) 233-245.

Williams, J, "Family presence during resuscitation: To see or not to see?" *Critical Care Nursing Clinics of North America* 37 (1) (2002) 211-220.

REFERENCES

1. P S Kidd, *Mosby's Emergency Nursing Reference* (St Louis: Mosby, Inc, 1996).
2. M Burke, "Disaster planning in the perioperative environment," in *Perioperative Services,* C Frye, C Spry, eds (Gaithersburg, Md: Aspen Publishers, 2002).
3. *Ibid.*
4. *Ibid.*

CHAPTER 16: PROFESSIONAL ACCOUNTABILITY

Rose Moss, RN, MN, CNOR

Professional accountability is inherent to the role of the professional registered nurse. However, accountability is a multi-faceted concept with varied interpretations. Every nurse is expected to practice nursing appropriate to one's education, experience, and position. The nurse is not only accountable to his/her patients, but also to peers and ultimately, one's self. In addition, there is a commitment between the nurse and society that he/she will demonstrate professional conduct based on a code of ethics and recognized standards of practice, such as state nurse practice acts; the American Nurses Association (ANA) *Code for Nurses with Interpretive Statements;* and the standards, recommended practices, and guidelines promulgated by AORN, the Association of periOperative Registered Nurses. The nurse also will take appropriate measures to maintain the specific knowledge and competencies required for one's specialty area of practice and actively seek opportunities for professional growth and performance improvement activities.

The perioperative environment is a highly specialized area that demands accountability in regard to collaboration and patient advocacy. The professional perioperative nurse practices in a unique milieu. Collaboration with other health care professionals, such as the surgeon, anesthesia care provider, and surgical technologist is a key element of quality patient care. Patient advocacy is another key component of professional nursing practice, as the patients are usually sedated and/or anesthetized. Therefore, ethical decision making is necessary when caring for surgical patients.

In today's dynamic health care environment and diversity in perioperative practice settings, critical thinking is a key element in professional accountability. Perioperative nurses must ask themselves whether they think critically. If the answer is no, the principles of critical thinking must be learned and applied in clinical practice. In addition, the nurse must critically examine the results of research studies and use them effectively to change practices for the ultimate good of the patient. This chapter will allow the perioperative nurse to assess his/her personal conduct and use the suggested learning activities and recommended study materials to develop and maintain professional accountability.

LEARNING OBJECTIVES

Professional registered nurses preparing for the certification exam in perioperative nursing should include the areas of requisite knowledge and skills to establish and maintain professional accountability. Upon completion of this chapter, the nurse should be able to:

1. Discuss the nursing responsibilities of professional accountability.
2. Identify the areas of knowledge and competency in nursing practice as they relate to professional accountability.
3. Describe the professional practice standards, regulations, and statutes that direct nursing practice.
4. State the nurse's responsibility for professional growth and performance improvement.
5. Define the elements of ethical decision making, critical thinking, collaborative practice, and research as they relate to positive patient outcomes.
6. Explain the impact of nursing research in improving perioperative nursing care.

TASK STATEMENT; AREAS OF KNOWLEDGE AND SKILL

Task Statement

The professional perioperative nurse performs nursing activities to demonstrate excellence in practice and contribute to the professional growth of the individual practitioner and the perioperative specialty.

Professional accountability includes the perioperative nurse's responsibility to incorporate professional standards and statutes into one's practice, provide ethical nursing care, develop critical thinking skills, and integrate research findings into practice to improve outcomes. Accountability also requires that the professional registered nurse recognize his or her learning needs, take the actions necessary for growth and development, contribute to the professional growth of colleagues and peers, and foster an environment of intellectual curiosity.

Areas of Knowledge

K-16 Emergency procedures (eg, CPR, MH)
K-21 Communication theories and techniques
K-25 *Perioperative Nursing Data Set* (PNDS)
K-37 Principles of product evaluation, cost containment, and resource management
K-39 Patient rights and responsibilities
K-40 Legal responsibilities and implications for patient care
K-42 Nursing research and evidence-based practice
K-43 "ANA Code of Ethics for Nurses with Explications for Perioperative Nurses"
K-44 Regulatory standards and voluntary guidelines
K-45 AORN *Standards, Recommended Practices, and Guidelines*
K-46 AORN position statements (eg, bloodborne pathogens, do-not-resuscitate orders [DNR])
K-47 Principles of problem solving
K-48 Quality improvement principles
K-49 Surgical consent laws and policies
K-58 Inappropriate workplace behaviors (eg, harassment, workplace violence)
K-53 Rules, responsibilities, and duties of health care team members, and internal and external support service personnel
K-55 Credentialing standards and clinical privileges
K-57 Health care trends and issues
K-58 Negotiation techniques
K-59 Opportunities for professional growth

Areas of Skill

S-4 Communicating effectively (verbal and nonverbal)
S-5 Advocating and protecting patient rights
S-16 Applying AORN *Standards, Recommended Practices, and Guidelines*
S-17 Applying the *Perioperative Nursing Data Set* (PNDS)
S-19 Participating in quality improvement activities
S-22 Providing evidence based care
S-23 Applying regulatory standards and voluntary guidelines
S-25 Apply principles of, and participate in, cost containment, product evaluation, and resource management
S-28 Adapting to changing situations and technologies
S-50 Adapting to special and unusual needs
S-53 Educating, mentoring, and supervising health care team members
S-54 Recognizing impaired behavior in patients, family, and staff and responding appropriately
S-55 Recognizing personal limitations and seeking assistance as needed
S-62 Setting priorities
S-63 Evaluating self and others according to goals and standards
S-64 Incorporating feedback into nurse performance
S-65 Applying ethical principles
S-66 Using resources for professional growth

PROFESSIONAL ACCOUNTABILITY

To fully understand and appreciate professional accountability in nursing practice, it is beneficial to review the evolution of nursing as a profession. By examining nursing from this perspective, the perioperative nurse can truly realize that nursing is a profession, rather than an occupation. The factors that differentiate a profession from an occupation include the following.

- A profession has a unique body of scientific knowledge. This knowledge is taught to those in the vocation through a specified training process. Nursing's unique body of scientific knowledge includes its language, norms, standards, symbols, and ethical behaviors taught in nursing education programs. Because nursing practice is dynamic, it can respond to an expanding knowledge base as a result of research activities. A good example of this expanding knowledge base is the development and use of the nursing process, especially the formulation of nursing diagnoses.

- The clients served by a profession trust the knowledge and judgment of the provider. Nursing has a societal agreement between the nurse and the client. Inherent in this agreement is that the nurse will provide care with competence and sound, educated judgment.
- A licensure process exists that dictates the scope of practice. Since 1938, state boards of nursing have mandated licensure and defined the scope of registered nursing practice.
- A code of ethics exists. The ANA has developed a "Code of Ethics for Nurses with Interpretive Statements" as the ethical code for the profession.
- A professional society exists to coordinate and advance the organization of the profession. The ANA is the professional society for registered nurses.

MAINTAINING KNOWLEDGE AND COMPETENCE

Perioperative nursing practice requires the practitioner to have a broad base of knowledge, manual skills, and the ability to effectively combine the two. As a professional, the perioperative nurse has an obligation to establish and maintain the appropriate level of knowledge, skills, and competency required for the care of the surgical patient.

The art and science of professional nursing practice involves both the behavioral and physical sciences, which are in a constant state of change and evolution. To function effectively in this environment and promote positive patient outcomes, the nurse must actively participate in ongoing continuing education and professional development. The professional nurse is accountable to both him/herself, as well as society, for this ongoing educational process. The methods by which the professional nurse can maintain knowledge and competence include the following.

- Orientation—including the identification of individual learning needs based on the specific competencies required in the practice setting.
- Professional development—setting goals and developing a plan to attain them.
- Performance criteria—using these criteria to judge competency.
- Continuing education—seeking continuing education opportunities to maintain a specific body of knowledge and current trends in a specialty practice area.

PROFESSIONAL PRACTICE STANDARDS, REGULATIONS, AND STATUTES

Practice standards, regulations, and statutes govern the practice of professional nursing. These various sets of guidelines exist to protect and promote the welfare of the patients that nurses serve. Accountability is a multi-faceted concept, which is sometimes described as the professional nurse's ability and willingness to foresee the results of one's actions, act accordingly, and be held accountable by one's peers. Therefore, the professional nurse is responsible for practicing within these guidelines. The following is a brief overview of the various regulations and guidelines that direct nursing practice.

- The ANA drafted its first model nurse practice act in 1915, and by 1923, all 48 states had enacted nursing licensure laws. Both the state's nurse practice act, and rules and regulations, usually referred to as administrative law, govern the practice of nursing for compensation. The legislature of each state is authorized to establish nursing licensure laws that are then enforced by the board of nursing. New legislation regarding nurse licensure is usually initiated through the state's nursing association or through the state board of nursing at the request of professional nursing organizations. The professional nurse's responsibilities are based on the ANA's *Standards of Clinical Nursing Practice* and the ANA's *Code for Nurses with Interpretive Statements.* The eight standards of professional performance, as outlined by the ANA, describe a competent level of behavior in the professional nursing role in the areas of quality of care, performance appraisal, education, collegiality, ethics, collaboration, research, and resource utilization. The ANA Code provides a context within which nurses can make ethically appropriate decisions for nursing care as well as the fulfillment of their responsibilities to the patient, other members of the health care team, and to the nursing profession.
- In 1982, the National Council of State Boards of Nursing, Inc. (NCSBN) developed a "Model Practice Act" to assist state boards of nursing in legally defining the scope of nursing practice. Currently, plans are in progress to revamp the

regulation of nursing practice from the single-state licensure model to a multistate licensure system. This model, called the "Mutual Recognition Model," has been proposed by the NCSBN in an effort to adapt nursing licensure to the dynamic transitions in today's health care environment.

- AORN, the Association of periOperative Registered Nurses, develops standards, recommended practices, and guidelines that provide a network of interrelated principles to guide nursing activities in the perioperative practice setting. Because the perioperative environment is changing so rapidly, these principles are stated in broad, flexible terms in order to adapt to the variety of practice settings. These standards, recommended practices, and guidelines are theory- and research-based and are updated and expanded on a regular basis, or as warranted by technological advancements.

- Other agencies assist the nursing profession in guiding and regulating practice. Two such organizations are the Occupational Safety and Health Administration (OSHA), which established guidelines for a safe work environment, and the Center for Disease Control and Prevention (CDC), which develops infection control standards.

The ever-changing health care environment reinforces the need for all nurses to stay informed of the current standards and statutes from regulatory agencies. This awareness directly affects the practice of nursing. Adherence to practice standards, regulations, and statutes is a key component of the nurse's commitment to society in maintaining accountability and responsibility for quality nursing care. Continual education and evaluation of nursing practice, according to the regulations, standards, and recommended practices, are vital factors in maintaining the autonomy of the nursing profession.

PROFESSIONAL GROWTH

As noted above, included in the defining characteristics of a profession is the responsibility of the nurse to implement and share knowledge of the standards, regulations, and statutes with colleagues and peers. In doing so, the professional nurse serves as the patient's advocate by providing safe and effective care. The ways the nurse can participate in professional growth initiatives include

- assisting colleagues in the practice setting to develop and maintain competencies;

- implementing changes in practice based on research findings;

- incorporating constructive feedback into safe and effective patient care practices; and

- protecting patients from colleagues who may be incompetent or unethical in their practice, such as working with colleagues who are impaired by drug or alcohol use; knowing about the performance of unethical procedures; or witnessing delegation of duties to staff members who do not have the education, experience, or licensure to carry out such functions.

PERFORMANCE IMPROVEMENT

The performance improvement process is continual in health care facilities today. It requires both input and feedback from the professionals directly involved with patient care—the nurse. Therefore, the perioperative nurse must comprehend the basic principles of performance improvement, appreciate his/her role related to specific performance improvement activities, and be willing to assume new and different practice patterns.

The performance improvement process requires a commitment from the health care organization, which is filtered throughout all departments and levels of caregivers. Continuous quality improvement is defined as the combination of principles and methods that create both a quality and customer focused environment as well as the capability to identify, assess, and constantly enhance the efficiency and effectiveness of those processes that determine significant organizational results. Performance improvement activities are most successful when they involve all staff and when departmental barriers are minimized or eliminated. The key principles of performance improvement follow.

- Continual improvement is the principal priority of the organization's mission and of daily activities.

- The organization's leaders are committed to and involved in the process (ie, they drive the process and provide the necessary resources).

- The primary focus is on the functions that influence outcomes; it is necessary to improve work processes, not just solve problems.

- Data are available and used in the decision-making process, including feedback from customers. In addition, the information system should support ease of data collection, entry, retrieval, and analysis.

- All staff members are held personally responsible for the performance improvement process by having control over their own performance, reducing internal barriers, and supporting a multi-disciplinary approach to process improvement.

- Everyone in the organization continually focuses on "doing better."

In today's dynamic health care environment, ensuring quality patient care and satisfaction, as well as implementing performance improvement measures, are key elements in the delivery of cost-effective, efficient care. The perioperative nurse has an obligation to be knowledgeable of and participate in both departmental and organization-wide performance improvement activities. The perioperative nurse must understand the principles of quality and performance improvement and data collection and analysis methods, and also actively participate in the process by providing input and feedback.

ETHICAL PATIENT CARE

Ethical decision making is a significant component of perioperative nursing practice, as perioperative nurses make ethical and advocacy decisions on a daily basis. Perioperative nurses must recognize ethical dilemmas and take action based upon the ethical code outlined in the ANA's *Code of Ethics for Nurses with Interpretive Statements*. A key element of ethical care is the protection of patients' rights, in addition to the right to safe care and competent practitioners. As the patient's advocate, the professional nurse uses practice standards to protect the health, safety, and rights of the patients. The need for patient advocacy results from the impact of illness on the patient's autonomy and his/her ability to make decisions. The following points outline the role of the nurse in providing ethical patient care.

- Practitioners are responsible for safeguarding patients' confidentiality and modesty. In the perioperative setting, this may include limiting access to the OR schedule; confining conversations about the patient to the OR suite and keeping them confidential; and minimizing patient exposure during positioning and skin preparation.

- Nurses must ensure that health care is provided without regard to race, sex, sexual preference, creed, or cultural beliefs.

- Care must be provided to the patient and significant others by including them in the decision-making process as well as respecting the patient's autonomy, dignity, and right to have input into his/her plan of care.

- Nurses may be placed in a difficult situation and need outside assistance to formulate an ethical plan of care with the patient. Examples of outside resources include the ethics committee, spiritual advisors, and social services.

The ethical protection of the surgical patient is the responsibility of all members of the perioperative team. As the first-line care taker of the patient, it is imperative that the perioperative nurse practice as the patient advocate at a time when the patient is often unable to protect him/herself due to the effects of anxiety, anesthesia, sedation, and the surgical experience itself.

CRITICAL THINKING

As previously discussed, the practice of professional nursing practice involves the establishment and continual refinement of a unique body of knowledge. As the profession has matured, a key component of this process was the introduction of the nursing process, defined as the steps of assessment, diagnosis, planning, implementation, and evaluation in the delivery of nursing care to help meet patients' needs. A vital element in the effective application of the nursing process is critical thinking.

Critical thinking is often associated with critical judgment in practice. While these terms are not synonymous, the application of critical thinking is most apparent in the decision-making process of clinical judgment. Critical thinking is usually defined as a domain-specific, disciplined thought process, which is autonomous and unique to every nurse. Other elements in the definition of critical thinking include that it is focused on deciding what to do; includes a tolerance for ambiguity; and involves the use of facts, principles, theories, and abstractions and interpretations.

The surgical environment is a unique practice area in which the perioperative nurse uses the nursing process, relative to the specific personnel, technology, and pharmacodynamics, to achieve very specific patient outcomes; therefore, critical thinking skills are crucial. The issue of patient safety in the surgical environment is often one of the implementation of measures that require critical thinking. Nurses must constructively question every perioperative patient care process and the ramifications of changing existing policies and practices. Perioperative nurses must actively hone their cognitive skills, learn to think critically, and base nursing actions on conclusions supported by research.

COLLABORATIVE PRACTICE

While professional nursing practice generally is considered a collaborative practice, nowhere is this more evident than in the perioperative setting. Reference is often made to the "surgical team," which truly is an interdisciplinary team of professional health care providers. The collaboration of all team members is essential for the best possible patient outcomes. There are four major components for collaborative practice to be successful.

- *Communication*—This is perhaps the most important component. In order to communicate clearly, the main objective must be stated clearly, so that each member of the team understands the individual concerns and responsibilities relative to accomplishing the objective.

- *Accountability*—Through accountability, the perioperative nurse assists other members of the surgical team to become aware of their respective roles. Once the roles are defined, the expectations of each member are established, thereby allowing the team to effectively use their specific areas of expertise toward achieving the goal.

- *Competence*—Competence builds respect and therefore increases cooperation.

- *Trust*—Trust is essential, but often difficult to establish unless all members listen and exchange information, accept and acknowledge everyone's specific role, and respect the individual practice area.

Once the collaborative practice process has begun, it is continuous. It links with the performance improvement process and focuses on providing the patient with the best possible care, using the collective expertise of the team. Through collaboration, the perioperative nurse combines his/her efforts with those of the other team members to address concerns such as safety, effectiveness and efficiency of care, and the implementation of appropriate nursing interventions.

NURSING RESEARCH

The research process always begins with a problem. Specifically, research in nursing practice begins with problems encountered in the practice setting. There is no paucity of clinical nursing problems, especially in the perioperative environment. With the diversity of practice settings and the expanding nursing role, it becomes more important than ever that nurses recognize the role of research in analyzing clinical problems for the ultimate goals of improved patient care, positive outcomes, and the advancement of the professional perioperative nursing practice.

The advancement of professional practice depends on the continuous development of the existing knowledge base. Nursing practice research means research on problems in patient care—that is, those issues that deal directly with nursing practice. Research provides the scientific basis for the credibility for the current standards and practices, as well as to support changes in practice patterns.

Once a problem has been identified and is recognized as a significant discrepancy, it must be converted into a form that will make it researchable. The steps in this process are

1. identify and state the discrepancy;

2. describe the significance of the discrepancy to theory and practice;

3. analyze the nature of the discrepancy;

4. state the questions the need to be resolved; and

5. specify the appropriate type of study.

After the problem is deemed worthy to be studied, the research process begins. Research studies have five basic components, as follows.

- *Problem*—This is a statement that clearly identifies the problem that will be studied, what the significance of the study will be, and what is already known about the problem. The research statement provides the theoretical background and a framework in which to view the problem.

- *Research methodology*—This is the description

of the study and how it will be conducted. Included in this description are the research design (eg, historical, descriptive, experimental); definition of the independent and dependent variables; methods for sample selection; data collection procedures; and the statistical tests that will be used for data analysis.

- *Objective findings*—These are reported either in a narrative format or as a combination of narratives and data in the form of graphs and/or charts.

- *Implications of the findings*—These include any limitations of the study or additional information gained during the research process. These implications also should relate the findings to previous research studies and should include the significance of the findings for practice.

- *Recommendations for future research*—These include additional areas related to the original study that need to be examined.

It is imperative that the professional perioperative nurse be aware of the role that research plays in nursing practice. While every nurse may not formally participate in the research process, it is important that the nurse

- reads current research articles related to practice issues,
- interprets research findings as they relate to practice,
- participates in the steps of the research process, as applicable,
- recognizes clinical problems that are amenable to the research process, and
- applies the knowledge from research studies to daily practice (eg, explaining policies and procedures, using as a basis for changing practice as appropriate).

The ultimate goal of any profession is to improve the practice of its members, so that the services provided to its clients will have the greatest impact. Any profession seeking to enhance its professional image and services undertakes the continual development of its body of knowledge that is fundamental to its practice. This continual refinement of such a body of scientific knowledge is vital in fostering a sense of both commitment and accountability to the recipients of nursing care. In today's dynamic health care environment, consumers of health care demand that professionals examine the efficacy of their practice and determine what impact their knowledge and skills have on society. While not every nurse can be a nurse researcher, every nurse can incorporate research findings into daily perioperative nursing practice. In doing so, nurses contribute to the body of scientific knowledge of perioperative nursing and thereby the expanding the scientific base of the nursing profession.

SUMMARY

Establishing and maintaining accountability are essential components in both the professional and personal growth of the perioperative registered nurse. The key components in accountability in professional nursing practice include

- maintaining knowledge and competence;
- incorporating professional practice standards, regulations, and statutes into daily nursing practice;
- supporting the professional growth of self, peers, colleagues, and other health care professionals;
- participating in and evaluating performance improvement activities;
- recognizing ethical dilemmas and taking appropriate action;
- developing and enhancing critical thinking skills;
- developing a collaborative approach to perioperative nursing care; and
- incorporating nursing research activities and findings into the role of the professional nurse.

There are many ways to demonstrate professional accountability in nursing practice. One of the best ways to exemplify accountability is to become certified in perioperative nursing. Successful completion of the certification exam is evidence of an increased level of knowledge and skill in perioperative nursing practice. In today's dynamic perioperative environment and diversity of practice settings, the perioperative nurses must continually update and maintain the necessary level of knowledge and skills to meet their responsibilities to their patients and society to provide quality nursing care and promote positive patient outcomes.

CASE STUDIES

Case Study: Ms. J, RN, CNOR

Ms. J, an agency nurse, is assigned to the scrub role in your room. You are setting up for a laparoscopic-assisted vaginal hysterectomy (LAVH). While you and Ms. J are setting up the room, you notice that Ms. J has brightly-colored artificial nails, is wearing a pearl necklace over her scrub top, and has long earrings dangling outside her scrub cap. You know that this attire is incorrect and that your facility policy clearly outlines proper attire. You approach Ms. J to explain this to her.

Points to Consider

- What knowledge is Ms. J lacking in regard to proper OR attire?
- What professional recommended practices outline appropriate OR attire?
- Does nursing research address jewelry in the OR?
- What is the impact on the patient?

Discussion of Points to Consider

- What knowledge is Ms. J lacking in regard to proper OR attire?
  She lacks the knowledge in the areas of:
  - AORN "Recommended Practices for Surgical Attire," which state, "All personnel entering the semirestricted and restricted areas of the surgical suite should confine or review all jewelry and watches; artificial nails should not be worn;"
  - infection control practices and methods of microbe transmission; and
  - facility policy regarding OR attire.
- What professional recommended practices outline appropriate OR attire?
  AORN "Recommended Practices for Surgical Attire"; facility-specific policies outlining surgical attire.
- Does nursing research address jewelry in the OR?
  Yes, the AORN "Recommended Practices for Surgical Attire" are based on the findings from applicable research studies. For example, one research study found that rings, watches, and bracelets may harbor organisms that cannot be removed during handwashing. This supports the recommendation that all jewelry should be removed in the semirestricted and restricted areas of the surgical suite. Another study found that fungal growth occurs frequently under artificial nails as a result of moisture trapped between the artificial and natural nails; this supports the recommendation that artificial nails should not be worn in the OR. A review of the bibliography provides supporting research studies used in the revisions of the recommended practices. The incorporation of AORN recommended practices into facility policies and procedures is a means of participating in the nursing research process.
- What is the impact to the patient?
  The impact to the patient is the increased risk for a potential postoperative surgical wound infection, resulting from the transmission of microbes. In addition, there also is a concern that jewelry, if not contained, could fall into the sterile field or wound itself. The necklace could contaminate the front of the sterile gown.

Case Study: Mr. R, CRNA

Mr. R has been practicing anesthesia for 8 years in the same hospital. Mr. R has always been very conscientious in his practice (ie, conducting thorough preoperative patient interviews, setting up his equipment early, and collaborating with all members of the perioperative team). During the past 6 months, you and other staff members have noticed a change in Mr. R's behavior: he frequently comes to work "just-in-time," and even late on some occasions; he has become increasingly impatient with both patients and other staff members; and he sometimes appears distracted during longer cases. In addition, the postanesthesia care unit (PACU) nurses are reporting that Mr. R's patients are requiring more pain medication than in the past. Today, you are assigned to a right hemicolectomy and Mr. R is the assigned anesthetist. You notice midway through the case that he has his head down on the anesthesia machine and appears to be asleep.

Points to Consider

- What is the risk to the patient?
- Whom must you advocate for and protect in this situation?
- What should you do?

Discussion of Points to Consider

- What is the risk to the patient?
  The obvious risk to the patient is the potential for an adverse reaction to anesthesia due to the impairment of the anesthetist.
- Whom must you advocate for and protect in this situation?
  In this situation, you should protect both the

patient and Mr. R. The obvious risk for the patient's safety, as noted above, is present when he/she is under the care of an impaired anesthetist. You also have an obligation to Mr. R to report the incident to his supervisor in order to help him get assistance and continue his practice and career.

- What should you do?
  The risk must be removed from the patient. You must report your observations immediately to the anesthesiologist supervising Mr. R for intercession in order to protect the patient. You should also report the situation to your manager, or appropriate administrator, as the situation has ramifications for the facility. The anesthesiologist must take appropriate action for the patient's welfare by removing Mr. R from the care environment and taking over the administration of anesthesia or provide another anesthetist. Perioperative nurses should be aware of programs that offer support to staff members in dealing with substance abuse problems.

SUGGESTED LEARNING ACTIVITIES

As a continuation of the self-assessment process, the following activities may be helpful in increasing your level of expertise regarding establishing and maintaining professional accountability in perioperative nursing practice.

◆ Obtain and read a copy of your state's nurse practice act. This document outlines the legal definition and scope of nursing practice in your state. Also read the OSHA and CDC recommendations and relate them to your practice setting.

◆ Obtain and review the ANA *Code for Nurses with Interpretive Statements.* Relate the code to your nursing practice and set goals to improve any areas in which you may feel are needed.

◆ Review the current AORN *Standards, Recommended Practices, and Guidelines.* Particularly note which areas are new and revised, and those areas in which you may need additional knowledge or skills.

◆ Read a pertinent research article in a professional nursing journal at least once a month. Describe the type of research study, its components, as well as its implications for nursing practice.

◆ Volunteer to be a member of your department's performance improvement committee/team to gain a better understanding of the performance improvement process and your role in it. Examine your practice area to identify a problem and work actively to resolve it, using the performance improvement process.

◆ Describe one area in your practice in which you can help a colleague or peer to increase his/her knowledge base. Further identify the best method by which to provide the information, then ask the colleague to provide feedback in evaluating your effectiveness.

◆ Challenge yourself to improve your critical thinking skills.

◆ Collaborate effectively with your coworkers, especially when in a conflict situation. Think of the elements of collaboration, communication, accountability, competency, and trust.

◆ Discuss ethical issues in the perioperative environment (eg, do-not-resuscitate orders, impaired coworkers) with a member of your facility's ethics committee. Discuss how the perioperative nurse assists the patient and significant others in ethical decision making and how the perioperative nurse makes his/her own ethical decisions. Report the feedback to your coworkers.

RECOMMENDED STUDY MATERIALS

AORN, *Standards, Recommended Practices, and Guidelines* (Denver: AORN, Inc, 2002).

American Nurses Association, *Code of Ethics for Nurses with Interpretive Statements* (Washington, DC: American Nurses Association, 2001).

Baker, C R, "Reflective learning: A teaching strategy for critical thinking," *Journal of Nursing Education* 35 (January 1996) 19-22.

Ellis, J R; Hartley, C L, *Nursing in Today's World: Challenges, Issues, and Trends,* sixth ed (Philadelphia: Lippincott Raven, 1998).

Gabel, R A; et al, *Operating Room Management* (Boston: Butterworth-Heinemann, 999).

Garner, J S, *Guidelines for Prevention of Surgical Wound Infection* (Atlanta: US Department of Health and Human Services, Public Health Service, CDC, 1985).

Koch, F T; Speers, A T, "It is time to move from the nursing process to critical thinking," *AORN Journal* 66 (August 1997) 318-320.

Meeker, M H; Rothrock, J C, eds, *Alexander's Care of the Patient in Surgery,* 12th ed (St Louis: Mosby, Inc, 2002).

National Council of State Boards of Nursing (US), Nursing Practice and Education Committee, *Model Nursing Practice Act* (second revision) (Chicago: National Council of State Boards of Nursing, Inc, 1994) 4.

OSHA, *Enforcement Procedures for the Occupational Exposure to Bloodborne Pathogens* CPL2-2.44D (Washington, DC: Occupational Safety and Health Administration, Nov 5, 1999).

OSHA, "Occupational exposure to bloodborne pathogens: Final rule," *Federal Register* 56 (Dec 6, 1991) 64175-64182.

Otto, D A, "Regulatory statutes and issues—clinical accountability in the perioperative setting," *AORN Journal* 70 (August 1999) 241-252.

Owen, S A, "Clinical exemplar demonstrates critical thinking and assertive perioperative nursing intervention," *AORN Journal* 65 (February 1997) 444-447.

Reavis, C W; Sandidge, J; Bauer, K, "Critical thinking's role in perioperative patient safety outcomes," *AORN Journal* 68 (November 1998) 758-772.

Schroeter, K, "Advocacy in perioperative nursing practice," *AORN Journal* 71 (June 2000) 1207-1222.

Schroeter, K, "Ethics in perioperative practice—patient advocacy," *AORN Journal* 75 (May 2002) 941-949.

Tanner, C A, "Rethinking clinical judgment," in *Transforming RN Education: Dialogue and Debate,* Diekelmann, N; Rather, M, eds (New York: NLN Press, 1993) 18-21.

Trauner, L, "It is time to move from the nursing process to critical thinking," *AORN Journal* 67

CHAPTER 17: STRATEGIES FOR SUCCESS:

GETTING PREPARED AND BEING TEST-WISE

Julia M. Leahy, RN, PhD, and Linda D. Waters, RN, PhD

Being successful in passing the CNOR certification examination for perioperative nursing requires having a sound foundation of the requisite knowledge and skills important for expert clinical practice and a thorough understanding of the test taking process.

Knowledge is attained through experience and formalized educational programs of study. The experiential knowledge component requires that an individual who is eligible to take the CNOR certification examination has a minimum of two years of experience in perioperative nursing. The knowledge component is acquired through a variety of learning activities, including formal education, self-study, and continuing education programs. It is the combination of experiential and cognitive knowledge that forms the foundation of expert clinical practice.

In addition to this evidenced-based clinical knowledge, you also will need to have a firm understanding of the testing process. There is a definite skill in answering multiple-choice test questions, and becoming familiar with these techniques will improve your chances of success.

This chapter provides information about planning a personalized study program, obtaining the necessary resources to assist in the preparation, understanding the processes involved with answering multiple-choice test questions, and developing sound test-taking strategies for being successful on your certification examination.

LEARNING OBJECTIVES

Upon completion of this chapter, you will:

1. Identify specific content areas in which you will need further knowledge.
2. Develop an action plan for pursuing the additional knowledge.
3. Identify resources that will be of assistance in preparing for the certification examination.
4. Identify the major components of multiple-choice test questions.
5. Develop skill in applying test-taking strategies when answering multiple-choice test questions.
6. Plan a success-oriented action plan for taking the certification examination.

DEVELOPING GOOD STUDY HABITS

Making the initial decision to take a certification examination is an important decision. For most test takers, becoming certified in a specialty nursing area accomplishes both personal and professional goals. The personal goal is a feeling of accomplishment—tackling a task that may be difficult yet, at the same time, rewarding. Professionally, certification provides external recognition of excellence in nursing and may promote career advancements.

The next step in the certification process is determining what your personal investment will be in preparing for the examination. And, what a personal investment it is! The easiest part is paying the examination fee. The more difficult part is determining realistically what you *want* to do and *can* do to prepare for the examination.

Use the following questions to determine what your personal investment in your certification examination will be.

Question #1 — Should I study for the examination?

Studying for the examination is your choice and is, in no small way, a decision based on your years of experience in perioperative nursing. While experience is critical, your personal work experiences may not have provided the broad skills and knowledge needed to be successful on the certification examination. Remember, a certification examination is a general examination that will ask questions about many areas of perioperative nursing. Ask yourself whether your experiences in perioperative nursing have been sufficiently broad enough to prepare you for all content areas possible.

So, do you need to study? Conduct a self-assessment to determine your chances of passing the certification examination.

How do you do that?

An excellent starting point is to review critical documents, including the CNOR Job Analysis and the AORN *Standards, Recommended Practices, and Guidelines.* For each content area that is identified, assess your "comfort level" with the area. Use a rating scale such as the one below to determine what you believe to be your level of competency:

1—*Very Certain:* I know this content area well and feel that my work experiences have fully prepared me.

2—*Certain:* I am reasonably comfortable with this content area and feel that my work experiences have prepared me reasonably well.

3—*Undecided:* I have some knowledge and some experiences in this area but there may be some content areas where I have a weakness or for which my work experiences have not fully prepared me.

4—*Uncertain:* I am aware that I have some knowledge deficits and/or lack work experience in this content area.

5—*Very Uncertain:* I am aware that I have many knowledge deficits and/or lack work experiences in this content area.

Then apply this rating scale to each area of the CNOR Job Analysis. Be honest with your self-assessment. If you rate all areas as "1s" or "2s," you may find that you will need little to no preparation before taking the examination. If, on the other hand, you find that you have a mixture of responses—some "1s" and "2s" along with some "3s," "4s," or "5s," you may find it very useful to develop a study plan for yourself.

Knowing that you have done all you can to prepare for taking the CNOR will provide you with that extra boost of confidence!

Be realistic! Preparing for the examination will be best completed over a period of weeks, not days or hours. Don't shortchange yourself. Allow sufficient study time before the examination.

Question #2 — What should I study?

Go back to the self-assessment you completed when making the decision whether to study. Consider dividing the content areas from the Job Analysis into three broad areas:

Area 1—Content that I have knowledge strengths

Area 2—Content that is mixed: I may know some areas but have weaknesses in others

Area 3—Content that I know I have knowledge weaknesses.

Then look at the proportion of the test that is dedicated to each area you identified. Concentrate your study time on those areas of the Job Analysis where you have the greatest knowledge weaknesses and where the largest percentage of test questions will be drawn. Tackle those needs FIRST before going on to other areas.

Question #3 — What is the best study style for me?

When you have decided that you do want to study for the examination and you have developed a study plan specific for your needs, next determine a study style that works best for you. Remember back to your school days. What worked best for you then? Were you more successful when you studied alone in the privacy of your own study space? Or were you more focused when you studied with others? Maybe a combination study style works best for you—individual study for reviewing familiar concepts and group study for learning new content areas.

What will likely be different now from your earlier study experiences in high school or college is the amount of time you have available for study. Looking back, those earlier days were a lot easier when you had fewer commitments. As you prepare for your certification examination, you must balance your other commitments (eg, family, work) with your need to prepare for your examination.

Plan the best time for taking the examination. If you know that the next few months are especially busy for you with unusual work expectations (eg, staff shortages, preparing for an accreditation visit) or family responsibilities (eg, vacation, child care), don't add to these burdens by scheduling the examination. Because the CNOR examination is available on a daily basis, choose to register for the examination at a time that is best for you—a time that allows you adequate preparation.

Remember, this certification examination is important for you both personally and professionally. Once you have made the commitment to take the examination, commit also to developing a personalized study plan—and stick to it!

Question #4 — How do I plan and manage my study time?

Once you have completed your self-assessment and identified what you need to study, you will be able to develop a study schedule that, if adhered to, should provide you with a successful outcome. Obviously, the more knowledge weaknesses you identify in major areas that will be covered on the CNOR examination, the greater time you will need to allow for fulfilling your study schedule.

Most important is to stay focused and committed to your study plan. You will be more confident if you plan for your study time and stick to the study schedule you develop.

Use your study time wisely. Make use of any spare time that you have to review concepts. Consider the following suggestions.

- Consider making flashcards out of index cards and carry them with you everywhere. That way, even an extra five minutes can be turned into valuable study time.
- Develop a note-taking system from your study periods. That way, you'll have a record of what areas you have reviewed and areas still outstanding.
- Color-code your notes according to their importance for the content area on the examination. In that way, if you have only a short amount of time to study one day, you can go right to the notes of greatest importance.

Question #5 — What do I study?

There are many excellent sources for study materials. Most importantly, be sure to review important AORN documents. The *AORN Journal* is an excellent resource for the latest knowledge in perioperative nursing. Because the timelines for printing journals are much shorter than textbooks, use journals as the source for new developments and important changes in nursing practice.

A second important source for review will be the "classic" textbooks in perioperative nursing. Look to see what textbooks are frequently cited in the literature or are the textbooks that everyone refers to when questions arise. Plan to spend some time reviewing these books. As you prepare for the CNOR examination, let these be your "best sellers" that replace novels.

Look to technology to provide a third source of study materials. There are excellent resources that can be found on-line or through the Internet. Consider combining your study preparation with earning continuing education credits. Complete continuing education programs that can be found on-line or simply call up a topic of interest and search the Internet to see what is available.

STUDY TIPS

As you plan your study, refer to the following handy study tips.

- *Study everyday—even if the best you can mange is a few minutes.* Studying every day helps you stick with your commitment to prepare for the examination and will help you feel a sense of accomplishment.
- *Balance "old" learning with "new" learning.* As you prepare for the examination, you will find some content areas where you need to simply review or "brush up" on your knowledge. In other cases, you may discover "new" content areas that you will need to learn. Remember that the examination is a general examination in perioperative

nursing, and the content areas evaluated by the examination may include areas that you have not previously worked in. Try to balance your study sessions to allow some new knowledge gains along with the review of more familiar content.

- *Use your work setting as your personal learning center.* In some ways, each workday provides you with an excellent opportunity to prepare for the examination. See how you can build in new knowledge in your daily activities. For example, are you administering a drug that is not used frequently? Use that opportunity to go to a reference and learn more about the drug. Are you assisting in a surgical procedure? Ask questions of your colleagues and find out all you can.

- *Let your work colleagues know that you are preparing for your certification examination.* Sharing your plans to take the certification examination with your work colleagues will accomplish two purposes.
  - First, ask them to "remind" you that you need to prepare for the examinations. Your colleagues can be a great source of support and encouragement. Give them the "okay" to ask you if you are on schedule with your preparation.
  - Second, ask your colleagues to become your study coaches. Remind them to seek you out when they have an interesting surgical case or when there is a new learning opportunity. You may want to share with your colleagues the areas where you believe you have knowledge weaknesses so they can be on the alert for work opportunities that relate.

- *Stay focused on your goal.* At some point in your study cycle, you will no doubt ask yourself, "Why did I decide to do this?" It's normal to feel a bit overwhelmed, but sticking to your goal will be rewarding.

COMPONENTS OF A MULTIPLE-CHOICE TEST QUESTION

In addition to a planned study program, you should develop your knowledge and skill in answering multiple-choice questions. It is important that you understand the structure and format of this type of test question.

The CNOR certification examination is composed of four-option multiple-choice test questions (or items). A multiple-choice test question consists of the stem and the options. The stem provides the information that supports the question that is being asked. It should contain sufficient information for you to understand what is being asked.

The stem is followed by four options, of which one is the correct answer (or key) as determined by a panel of content experts and current literature, and the other three options are the distracters, or wrong answers. There is one and only one best answer from the options provided. All questions are pretested to ensure that the question performs statistically as intended before being scored in an actual test form. One point is given for each correct answer. The total score on the examination is the total points given for all correct answers.

The stem of each test question may be closed-ended or open-ended. A closed-ended question asks a complete question and ends with a question mark. An open-ended question is a type of fill-in-the-blank with the four choices provided as the options. Each of the choices must complete the statement. The following are examples of each question format.

- Closed-end question:
  - Which of the following is the rationale for having perioperative nursing personnel immunized with hepatitis B vaccine?
    1. Current legislation requires the immunization.
    2. Occupational risk of acquiring the hepatitis virus is high.
    3. The immunization also provides protection against other forms of hepatitis.
    4. Universal precautions require routine immunization for all bloodborne viruses.

- Open-Ended Question:
  - Perioperative nursing personnel should receive hepatitis B immunization because:
    1. Current legislation requires the immunization.
    2. The occupational risk of acquiring the hepatitis virus is high.
    3. The immunization also provides protection against other forms of hepatitis.
    4. Universal precautions require routine immunization for all bloodborne viruses.

The multiple-choice test questions used in the CNOR examination measure either basic knowledge or facts or pose a situation in which an application of the knowledge is required. Because clinical practice requires the ability to apply principles and facts to patient situations, most of the test questions on the CNOR examination are at the application level. The following are examples of these two types of questions.

- Knowledge/Comprehension:
  - The loss of heat from exposed body parts due to exposure of air currents is known as:
    1. Evaporation.
    2. Conduction.
    3. Radiation.
    4. Convection.
- Application:
  - During skin preparation, the scrub person informs the perioperative nurse that the sleeve of a student's warm-up jacket has brushed against the area being prepared. Which of the following would be an appropriate response for the perioperative nurse to take first?
    1. Report the incident to the instructor for follow-up.
    2. Have the student review the required technique.
    3. Review skin preparation at the next inservice program.
    4 Inform the student immediately of the break in technique.

TAKING THE CNOR EXAMINATION

The CNOR examination is a computer-based test that is administered at a test center. Unlike paper-and-pencil tests where there may be several hundred individuals in the same room, the test center is designed to house about 10 to 15 computer stations and each person in the testing room may be taking a different examination. Some of these examinations may be shorter or longer than the CNOR examination, so you will notice that others either are leaving the room ahead of you or are still taking their examination when you have finished. You may find that some individuals are typing lengthy responses. If the noise is distracting, ask the proctor for ear plugs.

When the examination begins, you will first be given a 15-minute mandatory on-screen tutorial that will guide you in using the mouse to answer the test. While the mouse is more commonly used, the keyboard is enabled for use in answering questions. In addition, the tutorial will provide instructions on using the various features:

- "Previous," which allows you to return to a previously seen question;
- "Mark," which allows you to identify specific test questions that you would like to return to at a later time whether you have answered the question or skipped it; and
- "Review," which presents a list of all of the test questions and highlights those questions that you have marked. As you proceed through the test, you may skip a question and return to it later to answer. You may review questions at any time, not only at the end of the test.

You should complete the tutorial in its entirety, focusing on how the features of the test operate so that you are familiar with these functions. Your answers to the questions in the tutorial are not included in your test score.

The test center staff who proctor the examination and monitor your activities will be located in the room outside the testing room and are available if you need assistance. They are not content experts about perioperative nursing, so they are not able to provide you with any assistance about the test questions themselves. Their role is to monitor the activities in the testing room and report any unusual situations or inappropriate behavior. If you have a concern about a test question, you will have an opportunity to report your concern at the end of the examination.

You will find more information about the testing situation in the *CNOR Certification Recertification Policy Manual.* In addition, your Authorization to Test (ATT) letter includes instructions about the day of the examination, what time to arrive at the testing center, what identification you will need, and the name of the test you are taking.

HOW TO TAKE TESTS

For many individuals, the CNOR examination will be the first test taken in many years. The mere thought of sitting for more than four hours answering multiple-choice questions brings back memories of earlier, dreadful testing situations. So it is important that you prepare yourself to be in the best physical and mental condition possible.

Keep yourself in good physical health before the

examination date. You should plan to eat a balanced meal the evening before, and then get plenty of sleep. Plan to eat breakfast before a morning appointment (or lunch before an afternoon appointment), as you will be in the testing room for more than four hours. Avoid over-eating though, as too much food or liquids could make you tired. Feeling well and being rested is an important strategy for success. You need to be able to read carefully and think clearly.

Many people become anxious about the testing situation and have difficulty focusing and processing complex information. Mental anxiety stimulates the stress hormones, which have a direct impact on the cerebral cortex resulting in a decreased ability to think clearly and problem-solve. When this happens, you can become irritable and restless, be unable to sleep, and have difficulty thinking.

One way to reduce this anxiety is to desensitize yourself to the stressful situation. You can accomplish this by taking several practice tests and developing a sense of calm about the situation. As you feel better prepared, you will find that you can become less anxious. You also can engage in regular aerobic exercise and relaxation techniques, such as breathing exercises.

TEST-TAKING GUIDELINES

Being successful in passing the certification examination takes more than just knowing the content. You need to understand how to read and answer multiple-choice test questions. There is a very simple and easy-to-follow strategy in taking multiple-choice tests.

When reading multiple-choice test questions, it is important to remember that there is one and only one correct answer. So, consider the following.

- *Attempt to answer the question before reading the options, and then look for an option that best fits your answer.* You should be able to answer a good multiple-choice question without reading the options. Often you will find that your answer is one of the options provided. In that case, your best course of action is to go with your first answer.

- *Note that the options are written to be plausible to those who do not know the content.* Well-written multiple-choice questions are designed to have four plausible options. The intent is to discriminate between those candidates who know the information and those who do not. If you are unsure of the answer, try to eliminate options that you believe are incorrect. This improves your chance of selecting the correct answer.

- *Eliminate options that have absolutes, such as "always" or "never."* There is very little in nursing practice that is absolute. Most courses of action in clinical practice and most client responses are "usually" or "generally."

- *Read the question carefully, paying special attention to phrases, such as "most," "most appropriate," "primarily," "first," and "initially."* Often all of the options are applicable to the situation, but only one option fits the emphasis included in the stem.

- *Take careful note of phrases, such as "not," "least," or "except."* These words in the stem tend to confuse the reader, because the correct answer for the test question is the wrong response or the wrong thing to do.

- *Answer all of the questions.* Credit is given to all correct answers, and there is no penalty for selecting the wrong response. So if you are unsure of an answer, take an educated guess between plausible options.

- *Monitor your progress by noting the time remaining on the computer screen.* The CNOR examination is timed to provide you with about one minute per question. If you find that you are taking more time than usual to answer a question, mark the question and return to it when you have finished reading through the entire test. You don't want to spend too much time reading one test question and then run out of time, leaving several questions at the end unanswered.

- *Review your work after you have completed the test.* Once you have read through the test and answered as many questions as you can, you should first return to review the questions that you may have skipped or marked for further review. Then, if there is available time when you have completed the entire test, you can review all of the questions and reconsider your choices. You should refrain from making too many changes. Often, test takers change a right response to a wrong response.

HOW TO AVOID MAKING ERRORS

Being successful in passing the certification examination requires that you also avoid making mistakes in answering the test questions. One helpful strategy to avoid test-taking errors is to take practice tests. Become familiar with the format of multiple-choice questions. Use the practice tests as a method of improving your knowledge and identifying areas for further study.

When answering practice questions, consider the following as methods to avoid making testing errors.

- *Read each question carefully.* Errors are made when you don't read the question carefully. Look for and identify the important points involved with the question. Read each option carefully, noting which option most closely matches the intent of the question. Eliminate the options that are not plausible.

- *Assume that all of the information you need is presented in the test question.* The stem of a multiple-choice test question should contain all of the information that is necessary for the test taker to answer the question. When you read the question, avoid the common pitfall of "reading into" the question. Doing this may only confuse you. If certain patient characteristics, such as age, marital status, clinical setting, or other related information, are important to know to answer the question, then it is provided. Otherwise, answer the question from the perspective of the most common situation.

- *Identify content areas where your knowledge base is weak.* Use the practice test as an opportunity to evaluate your current knowledge of perioperative nursing. When you answer questions incorrectly, use the opportunity to learn the reasons for the incorrect answers. Ask yourself, "Why was my choice wrong?" The best way to learn the content is to understand the underlying rationale for the correct as well as the incorrect answers.

- *Understand the basic intent of the test question.* One of the most common errors that test takers make is not understanding the intent of the question. Is the question asking for you to make a decision about identifying a priority, a sequence of events, or an important patient phenomenon? Often in these types of questions, all of the options are plausible for the situation, but the correct answer is the one that is most important, has the highest priority, or is the first action to be taken. You should look for the clue words that give you the direction or emphasis to take.

DAY-OF-TEST CHECKLIST

Within 24 hours prior to the day of the examination, you should plan to follow this list of activities.

- *Avoid engaging in any known stressful events.* Many of us know what events tend to cause us stress. If at all possible, try to avoid engaging in or attending events that are known stressors just before taking the examination. Practice using relaxation methods to create a calm mental perspective about the test. This will minimize the production of stress hormones and enable you to think clearly and problem solve the questions.

- *Obtain sufficient rest and sleep.* Fatigue and lethargy will only inhibit your thinking and problem-solving abilities. Engage in any sleep rituals that tend to promote your sleeping ability.

- *Limit use of any stimulants, including coffee.* Stimulants will affect your ability to receive sufficient rest and sleep. Avoid taking any stimulants, including coffee, late in the day and before bedtime the night before the test.

- *Review the CNOR confirmation packet with regard to your responsibilities on the day of the examination.* It is your responsibility to be aware of the rules and regulations regarding the CNOR testing experience. If you do not follow the rules as outlined in the confirmation packet, you can be denied access to the testing center. After all of your studying and planning, you do not want to forfeit your testing opportunity at the last minute.

- *Arrive at the testing center at least 30 minutes prior to your test appointment.* If you are unsure of the exact location of the test center, it is highly-suggested that you locate the test center ahead of time. Determine how long it will take you to drive there or to go by public transportation, if applicable, by following the route before the day of your test. The test center can provide you with directions if you need them. On the day of the test, you should plan to arrive at the test center at least 30 minutes ahead of time. Unforeseen and uncontrollable events, such as accidents or inclement weather, can cause delays in your travel time. It is far better to be very early, then to be late and miss your appointment.

- *Bring few personal items with you.* You will not be permitted to take handbags, wallets, books, cellular phones, laptops, or any other personal belongings into the testing room. The test center has lockers where you can secure your valuables. You may take a pencil into the room, and the proctor will provide you with scrap paper.

- *Make sure that you bring the following items with you to the test center:*
  - Authorization to Test letter. This informs the test center staff of your eligibility to test, your name and the test that you are taking.
  - Two forms of identification, one of which must be a current, government-issued photo identification, such as a driver's license or a passport.
  - Watch.

SUMMARY

Being successful occurs when you have made a detailed plan for preparing for the examination and stick to it! Identifying knowledge areas for review, taking frequent practice tests, understanding the testing process, and getting yourself into the best mental state are essential components of success.

SUGGESTED LEARNING ACTIVITIES

As part of your action plan for success, you may consider some of the following learning activities helpful.

- Obtain a reference list of textbooks and/or journals that will provide you with the necessary information to expand your knowledge base of perioperative nursing.
- Begin studying those areas that you have identified as being your weak areas.
- Organize a study group of coworkers and other colleagues, if possible.
- Attend as many continuing education programs as are available.
- Practice taking multiple-choice test questions by answering the questions at the end of this study guide.

APPENDIX I:

PRACTICE QUESTIONS

1. Mr. G. is a 70-year-old man scheduled for a transurethral resection of the prostate under spinal anesthesia. One year ago, he underwent a left total hip replacement. Special precautions in caring for Mr. G. should include:
   1. Placing extra padding under the left buttock and adjusting the left stirrup lower than the right.
   2. Using caution in positioning him for the anesthetic and in placing his legs in the stirrups.
   3. Carefully positioning the left leg in the stirrup, maintaining an adducted position.
   4. Placing extra padding under the right buttock, and adjusting the right stirrup lower than the left.

2. During surgery on neonates, calculating blood loss by weighing sponges and carefully measuring suction bottle contents is especially important, because in infants:
   1. Weighing sponges provides a reliable means of judging the amount of blood lost.
   2. The need for blood replacement is established upon loss of 15% of total volume.
   3. Blood loss is replaced with 5% dextrose in lactated ringer's solution on an equal basis.
   4. The blood lost is replaced with an equal quantity of plasma expanders.

3. A female patient is scheduled for a cholecystectomy. While the perioperative nurse is assessing the patient's nutritional status, the patient tells the nurse that she has been on a crash diet, and has taken 3 diuretic tablets each day for the past 7 days. The nurse would review the collected data to determine if the patient's:
   1. Serum potassium level is below normal.
   2. Urine specific gravity is above 1.045.
   3. Serum sodium level is below normal.
   4. Weight loss has exceeded 30 lb (13.5 kg) in the past month.

4. When doing the preoperative skin preparation on an abdominal case, the perioperative nurse should start at the:
   1. Nipples and proceed toward the pubis.
   2. Site of incision to the periphery.
   3. Incision site and proceed upwards to nipples.
   4. Umbilicus and proceed in circles around it.

5. All personnel moving within or around a sterile field should do so with the goal of maintaining the sterile field. To best meet this goal, it is preferable that:
   1. All unscrubbed team members maintain a 6-inch distance from the sterile field and pass facing it.
   2. The scrub person stays close to the sterile field.
   3. All scrubbed team members pass each other face-to-back.
   4. All unscrubbed team members maintain a 12-inch distance from the sterile field and pass facing away from it.

6. Skin burns from the electrosurgical unit are most likely due to:
   1. Low skin resistance.
   2. High voltage.
   3. High current on a small area of contact.
   4. High leakage current.

7. During the preoperative assessment of a patient scheduled for a lumbar laminectomy, the nurse notes several inflammed pustules at the likely incision line. The most appropriate nursing action

would be to:
1. Advise the patient to bathe with povidone/iodine (Betadine).
2. Notify the surgeon.
3. Document the condition of the patient's skin.
4. Notify the preoperative holding nurse.

8. An inexperienced nurse who is a recent graduate is being assigned to cases in a busy OR that is understaffed due to vacations and illnesses. The graduate would be best utilized by being assigned to:
   1. Procedures performed by a surgeon known to be friendly and helpful to nurses.
   2. Procedures allowing an opportunity to work in close proximity to an experienced nurse.
   3. Procedures where the graduate is able to identify and meet patient needs.
   4. Perform preoperative assessments and postoperative evaluations.

9. A 20-year-old patient is admitted to the OR for exploratory laparotomy one hour after sustaining a gunshot wound to the lower abdomen. The circulating nurse's primary concern is to:
   1. Ensure that the surgeon and surgeon's assistants are available.
   2. Provide assistance to the anesthesiologist.
   3. Ensure that the scrub person has all the necessary supplies.
   4. Provide adequate supplies of blood and other IV fluids.

10. A patient's preoperative assessment reveals current electrolyte values of sodium = 136 mEq/L, potassium = 2.8 mEq/L, and chloride = 101 mEq/L. On the basis of these data, the perioperative nurse should:
    1. Inform the anesthesiologist.
    2. Send a sample to the laboratory for repeat electrolyte analysis.
    3. Check the complete blood count to correlate the hematocrit with these electrolyte results.
    4. Recognize that these electrolyte values are normal.

11. The manufacturer's directions for flash-sterilizing an arthroscope state that the item must be wrapped loosely in a towel. Which of the following procedures complies with basic principles of sterilization?
    1. Place in a tray without other instruments and flash-sterilize for 3 minutes at 270° F.
    2. Sterilize in a gravity displacement sterilizer for 10 minutes at 270° F.
    3. Soak in 2% activated glutaraldehyde for 20 minutes.
    4. Place in a sterilizer tray lined with towels and flash-sterilize for 20 minutes at 270° F.

12. An operating room supervisor arrives on duty and is informed that the humidity in the operating room stands at 95%. The individual room closets are well supplied with sterile linens and paper-wrapped packages, but all packages are damp to the touch. The supervisor should first:
    1. Obtain fresh sterile supplies and proceed with the daily schedule.
    2. Delay all elective surgical cases until the humidity problem is corrected.
    3. Request the assistance of central supply in replacing all contaminated supplies.
    4. Ask engineering to raise the room temperature to reduce the moisture content of the room air.

13. Constant monitoring and documenting of the temperature of a pediatric patient is essential during the intraoperative period because:
    1. Significant heat loss can occur from exposure of the child.
    2. Anesthesia may cause vasoconstriction and an increase in body temperature.
    3. A sudden decrease in temperature is indicative of the need for fluid replacement.
    4. A wide range of temperature variations is usually indicative of serious complications.

14. The appropriate time to position the anesthetized patient is when the:
    1. Anesthesia provider indicates that the patient can be moved.
    2. Entire surgical team is available and ready to begin surgery.
    3. Room setup is complete and all needed equipment is present.
    4. Surgeon is ready to begin and sufficient help is available to accomplish the positioning.

15. A primary concern for a nurse preparing the OR for surgery on an infant is initiating measures to:
    1. Maintain proper body alignment.
    2. Prevent loss of body heat.
    3. Ensure that all supplies are assembled before the patient arrives.
    4. Ensure that the anesthesia staff is standing by.

16. The purpose of using longitudinal body rolls for

a patient in the prone position is to:
1. Decrease abdominal pressure on the vena cava.
2. Prevent brachial and peroneal nerve damage.
3. Prevent circulatory depression.
4. Allow free chest and diaphragm expansion.

17. When evaluating sterile disposable suction tips for surgical use, consideration is given to all but one of the following:
   1. Type of sterilizing agent used.
   2. Cost of product.
   3. Methods of cleaning.
   4. Ease of package opening.

18. During the preoperative interview, a 38-year-old patient scheduled for a breast biopsy and a possible mastectomy states, "I know if I have a mastectomy tomorrow, my husband won't find me attractive anymore." In this situation, the nurse should:
   1. Encourage the patient to get a good night sleep before surgery.
   2. Mention ways of adjusting clothing to preserve normal body contours following mastectomy.
   3. Assure the patient that the mastectomy will not affect her relationship with her husband.
   4. Provide information about support group program options for mastectomy patients.

19. In the absence of a washer-sterilizer, which procedure should be used to clean instruments after a vascular procedure on a long-term hemodialysis patient?
   1. Soak in bactericidal solution for 20 minutes then flash-sterilize for 3 minutes at 270° F.
   2. Soak in phenolic solution for 20 minutes then hand-wash.
   3. Place in the ultrasonic cleaner.
   4. Rinse in water, then place in a perforated tray and flash-sterilize for 3 minutes at 270° F.

20. For a patient undergoing lumbar laminectomy in the prone position, the safest place to apply the dispersive electrode for the electrosurgical unit is the:
   1. Anterior thigh.
   2. Buttock.
   3. Posterior thigh.
   4. Calf.

21. During transport to the OR for an emergency appendectomy, a 13-year-old patient begins to cry, stating that she lied to the surgeon about intercourse and thinks she is pregnant. She asks that the nurse not reveal this information. The nurse's most appropriate response is to:
   1. Tell the parents, because they have signed a consent form with inadequate information.
   2. Document the conversation in the nurse's notes.
   3. Protect the patient's confidence, but inform the patient that the surgeon must be told.
   4. Tell the health care team members in the room.

22. The parent of a 5-year-old boy scheduled for a hernia repair reports that the child is extremely upset about having to remove his undershorts during surgery, and asks if the child can be allowed to wear cotton shorts. The nurse's most appropriate response would be to:
   1. Explain that the shorts must be removed to ensure that they are not lost during the procedure.
   2. Explain that removing the shorts is hospital policy that cannot be altered.
   3. Explain that removing the shorts is necessary to help prevent postoperative infection.
   4. Allow the child to wear the shorts.

23. An 11-year-old boy who has just arrived in the OR becomes curious about the anesthetic mask. The anesthesiologist begins to explain how the mask will be held over the patient's face. In this situation, the perioperative nurse might do all of the following except:
   1. Hold the patient's hand to provide reassurance.
   2. Continue to protect the patient during the induction phase.
   3. Allow the patient to hold the mask to his face.
   4. Stand by the bed and hold the patient so that he is immobilized.

24. The scrub nurse setting up for an emergency cesarean section examines the lap sponges on the back table and notes that no x-ray detectable strip is visible. The appropriate response in this situation is to:
   1. Make note of the missing strips on the operative record and proceed with the sponge count.
   2. Proceed with the sponge count in order to avoid delaying the start of the emergency procedure.
   3. Remove the lap sponges from the OR and obtain a new package for the set-up.
   4. Proceed with the count but have the circulating nurse obtain a second package.

25. During an operative procedure, metal instruments stored with rubber protective tips need to be sterilized. Which of the following methods, in a gravity displacement sterilizer, would the perioperative nurse use to sterilize these instruments?
    1. Remove the protective tips and sterilize for 10 minutes at 121.1° C (250° F).
    2. Remove the protective tips and sterilize for 3 minutes at 132.2° C (270° F).
    3. Leave the protective tips on and sterilize for 3 minutes at 121.1° C (250° F).
    4. Leave the protective tips on, place the instruments on a towel, and sterilize for 3 minutes at 132.2° C (270° F).

26. It becomes apparent to the surgical team that a patient does not want to have surgery, and the procedure is therefore canceled. The circulating nurse should:
    1. Document the situation on an incident report.
    2. Ask two other nurses to witness the incident.
    3. Call the risk manager for further instructions.
    4. Document the situation on the OR record.

27. Consideration when placing a patient in the Trendelenburg position includes all but:
    1. Venous stasis in the extremities.
    2. Drainage of secretions from lung bases.
    3. Increased intracranial pressure.
    4. Visceral pressure on the diaphragm.

28. As a cost-containment measure, a hospital is considering use of regular masking tape instead of indicator tape on in-house packaging of OR supplies. This change would not be advisable, primarily because:
    1. Masking tape has very strong adhesive properties, and will require extra time to remove.
    2. The adhesiveness of masking tape does not hold up under moisture during sterilization.
    3. Masking tape does not provide an external indicator of sterilization effectiveness.
    4. Chemical indicators will not function correctly if placed in a sterilizer along with packages sealed with masking tape.

29. A patient has received permission to wear a hearing aid until after induction. After induction, the perioperative nurse should:
    1. Label the hearing aid and have it delivered to the PACU, and inform staff there of the patient's dependence upon it.
    2. Leave the hearing aid in place so that the patient can hear upon awakening in the PACU.
    3. Put the hearing aid on the patient's transportation vehicle, so that it is available when the patient arrives in the PACU.
    4. Remove the hearing aid and have it picked up by the preoperative holding room nurse, so it will not be mislaid by OR personnel.

30. Which one of the following describes the proper application of a prone-positioning principle?
    1. When turning the patient, the head is appropriately supported with the neck in alignment with the spinal column.
    2. The breasts are supported by body rolls extending across the chest.
    3. The iliac crests rest on a pillow to increase abdominal pressure.
    4. The arms are supported on armboards with the elbows straight, and the hands supinated at either side of the head.

31. The bowie-dick test is used to determine which of the following?
    1. Proper functioning of an ethylene oxide (EO) sterilizer.
    2. Detect residual air in the chamber of a prevacuum sterilizer.
    3. Penetration of the sterilizing agent in a gravity displacement sterilizer.
    4. Correct temperature reached in a low-temperature gas plasma sterilizer.

32. A patient exhibits a dramatic drop in BP when her legs are lowered from the lithotomy position after a vaginal hysterectomy. This finding is most likely due to:
    1. Pooling of circulation in the splanchnic area masking an operative blood loss.
    2. Premature movement stimulating the pain reflex.
    3. Hemodynamic adjustment as blood shifts into the lower extremities.
    4. Bleeding induced by the change in pressure in the femoral area.

33. At the first sign of a negative reaction to a blood transfusion, the nurse should:
    1. Check the patient's vital signs.
    2. Notify the surgeon.
    3. Notify the PACU.
    4. Complete an incident report.

34. In the supine position, areas especially susceptible to skin breakdown include the:
    1. Occiput, the scapulae, and coccyx area.

2. Elbows, the ilium, and the back of the heels.
3. Knees, the back of the heels, and the brachial plexus.
4. Scapulae, the buttocks, and the clavicle.

35. An oral surgeon has requested that all procedures be supplied with ethylene-oxide sterilized lidocaine in single-dose vials. The request should be denied because:
    1. The oral cavity is contaminated, so there is no need to provide sterile cartridges.
    2. Local anesthesia of the oral cavity can be accomplished by using lidocaine from a multi-dose vial.
    3. The ethylene oxide may enter the solution through the rubber stopper.
    4. Ethylene oxide sterilization is not cost-effective for this procedure.

36. Which of the following actions would best prevent burn injuries resulting from use of the electrosurgical unit?
    1. Providing the surgeon with a foot-activated active electrode.
    2. Placing the active electrode tip on a moist sponge when it is not in use.
    3. Placing the active electrode tip in a container when it is not in use.
    4. Cleaning the active electrode tip with a sponge before each use.

37. During an exploratory laparotomy, the surgeon discovers a large abscess and a culture is taken. The perioperative nurse's best action would be to:
    1. Notify the supervisor of a dirty case.
    2. Keep the culture with the other specimens.
    3. Chart the organism suspected.
    4. Send the culture to the laboratory immediately.

38. A patient admitted through the emergency department is unconscious and has a diagnosis of possible ruptured abdominal aortic aneurysm. The nurse's first priority in preparing this patient for surgery would be to:
    1. Assemble supplies for an abdominal shave prep.
    2. Obtain a nasogastric tube for aspiration of stomach contents.
    3. Insert an indwelling urethral catheter with urimeter.
    4. Ensure availability of blood components and plasma expanders.

39. A patient undergoing a transurethral resection of the prostate (TURP) under spinal anesthesia starts to experience chest pain and restlessness with all the signs of congestive heart failure. The most likely cause is:
    1. Too high a level of anesthesia.
    2. An adverse reaction to the bladder being filled and emptied rapidly during surgery.
    3. Serum electrolyte imbalance.
    4. Systemic absorption of irrigation fluid into the vascular system.

40. A patient admitted through the emergency department has a deep scalp laceration and maxillary and cervical fractures. After evaluating the patient, the perioperative nurse's next action should be to:
    1. Prepare the fiberoptic laryngoscope.
    2. Apply pressure to stop bleeding from the laceration.
    3. Maintain head immobilization.
    4. Prepare for adequate suction.

41. A patient has undergone a partial right lobectomy. The primary concern of the perioperative nurse at the conclusion of the surgery is to:
    1. Provide appropriate equipment to secure the water-seal system to the floor.
    2. Ensure that the water-seal system is correctly assembled.
    3. Have large clamps available for clamping the chest tube.
    4. Have a syringe with a large-bore needle ready for air aspiration of the pleura.

42. During the preoperative assessment, a patient reports being unable to understand the scheduled procedure. The operative consent has been signed. The perioperative nurse's most appropriate action would be to:
    1. Explain the surgery and obtain a newly signed operative consent.
    2. Inform the surgeon that the consent has been signed without adequate knowledge and request that the surgeon speak with the patient about the procedure.
    3. Document the patient's response in the OR nursing care plan and inform the OR supervisor.
    4. Alert the OR supervisor that OR staff may be legally implicated in the lack of informed consent.

43. During an emergency procedure, the patient's condition becomes unstable and the surgeon

requests that no sponge count be performed. The immediate action of the circulating nurse would be to:
1. Inform the surgeon of hospital policy regarding sponge counts.
2. Instruct the scrub nurse to assist with the count.
3. Call the supervisor for instructions.
4. Document the omitted count.

44. A patient scheduled for a diagnostic D & C is not wearing an identification band when admitted to the OR. The patient is alert and states her name on request. The perioperative nurse's most appropriate action is to:
   1. Request that the surgeon identify the patient.
   2. Compare the signatures found on the informed consent and the admission sheets.
   3. Compare the patient's response to the chart information and obtain an identification band.
   4. Document the patient's response and proceed into the OR.

45. A patient being moved into the jackknife position should be placed with the:
   1. Face turned to the side and arms supported on armboards.
   2. Face down and arms outstretched on armboards.
   3. Face turned to the side and arms secured at sides.
   4. Face down and arms secured at sides.

46. Hypotension can occur following prolonged time in the lithotomy position. To minimize the possibility of this occurrence, the perioperative nurse should:
   1. Obtain padded knee support stirrups.
   2. Raise and lower both of the patient's legs simultaneously and slowly.
   3. Notify the postanesthesia care unit (PACU) of the position, to avoid undue concern.
   4. Keep dopamine intropin on hand in case the anesthesia provider should request it.

47. Concerning the transport of a patient with a compound fracture of the humerus to the operating room, the best description of the outcome goal is that the patient will be free of:
   1. Pain.
   2. Anxiety.
   3. Injury to joints adjacent to the injury.
   4. Further injury at the fracture site.

48. During an abdominal aortic aneurysmectomy, the perioperative nurse should be prepared to:
   1. Test the patient's urinary glucose and acetone.
   2. Monitor the patient's pedal pulses.
   3. Provide warmth to the patient's upper extremities and thorax.
   4. Check the patient's nail beds for cyanosis.

49. During a procedure, the surgeon asks the perioperative nurse to inform the family that the patient is not doing well. After providing the information to the family, the nurse's most appropriate next action would be to:
   1. Inform the surgeon of the family's reaction.
   2. Notify the organ procurement program of the anticipated death.
   3. Ask if the family wishes to have a member of the clergy notified.
   4. Notify the charge nurse that the next case will be delayed.

50. Considering the effects of anesthesia, prolonged cavity exposure, and an air-conditioned operating room, a perioperative nurse should assess a patient's total status with specific attention to:
   1. Maintaining patient comfort.
   2. Maintaining appropriate room humidity.
   3. Preventing shivering if the patient becomes cold.
   4. Preventing hemodynamic changes resulting from hypothermia.

51. To monitor for potential complications related to a craniotomy performed with the patient in the sitting position, the perioperative nurse should ensure availability of which of the following?
   1. Arterial line, EEG, EKG.
   2. Doppler, CVP line, left atrial line.
   3. Hypothermia unit, temperature probe.
   4. Blood gas kit, lumbar puncture tray.

52. A patient in hypovolemic shock is brought to the operating room for an emergency laparotomy. The nurses have not had time to perform an instrument count. The most appropriate course of action for the perioperative nurse to take would be to:
   1. Ask to have an x-ray taken prior to closure.
   2. Count at the conclusion of the surgical procedure and compare the count with the standard instrument list.
   3. Insist that the surgical procedure be delayed until the count is completed.
   4. Document that the instrument count has been omitted and state the reason.

53. After the repair of an abdominal aortic aneurysm, the surgeon requests that an aortogram be performed before the incision is closed. The perioperative nurse's immediate response would be to:
    1. Notify the radiology department of the request.
    2. Notify the OR supervisor of the request.
    3. Place any preoperative arteriograms on the radiology viewbox.
    4. Obtain methylene blue for the dye study.

54. The perioperative nurse observes that a surgeon has begun arthroscopy on the wrong knee and quickly informs the surgeon. After a lengthy pause, the surgeon resumes work on the same knee, while remarking, "Both knees needed to be scoped; I'll do the other one later." As a patient advocate, the nurse should:
    1. Support the surgeon's decision.
    2. Document the occurrence in an incident report.
    3. Communicate the occurrence to the chief of surgery.
    4. Inform appropriate administrative personnel immediately.

55. During a cervical laminectomy, the patient is in a sitting position with a skull pin headrest, when an air embolism occurs. In this situation, the most important measure the perioperative nurse can take is to:
    1. Contact the intensive care unit and ask if the unit can arrange to have a bed available postoperatively.
    2. Lower the head of the patient to reduce the angle of the position.
    3. Ensure that the scrub nurse has normal saline for the surgeon to irrigate the area.
    4. Advise the laboratory that blood gases will be sent soon and order a central venous pressure.

56. The nurse's initial response to a patient who develops signs of cyanosis during the preoperative assessment is to:
    1. Administer oxygen and start an IV line.
    2. Begin cardiopulmonary resuscitation.
    3. Read the history and physical to determine health status.
    4. Assess for breath sounds and airway obstruction.

57. If a sponge count is incorrect, the perioperative nurse should first:
    1. Arrange for an x-ray to be taken of the operative area.
    2. Document the incorrect count on the record.
    3. Notify the operating room supervisor.
    4. Notify the surgeon.

58. During the preoperative assessment, a patient adamantly states a desire to be told nothing about what will occur during surgery. The perioperative nurse should respond by:
    1. Presenting information with the patient's family present.
    2. Not forcing information on the patient.
    3. Giving the patient literature to read and leave the room.
    4. Leaving the patient's room to seek advice from the charge nurse.

59. A nursing diagnosis states the patient is free of signs and symptoms of injury related to positioning and length of surgical procedure. Which of the following outcome criteria would indicate that appropriate measures were taken?
    1. Orientation to name, date, and place.
    2. Ability to focus on objects 2 to 3 feet away.
    3. Equal bilateral breath sounds.
    4. Able to flex and extend all extremities.

60. Ms. M is to undergo an open reduction and internal fixation of her ankle. The surgeon requests the use of the pneumatic tourniquet. To prevent neurovascular damage, the perioperative nurse should apply the tourniquet cuff to the:
    1. Mid-calf area.
    2. Middle third of the thigh.
    3. Point of maximum circumference.
    4. Distal third of the thigh.

61. A hospital has recently installed new computerized flash sterilizers. These sterilizers produce a printout on which the conditions for sterilization are recorded. The perioperative nurse verifies that conditions for sterilization have been met:
    1. After the instruments have been placed on the back table.
    2. While the instruments are being removed from the sterilizer.
    3. While the sterilizer is in its sterilization cycle.
    4. Before the instruments have been removed from the sterilizer.

62. A commercially prepared item that has no expiration date and is labeled sterile unless the package integrity is violated should be:

1. Used, if package integrity has not been compromised.
2. Retained unused and returned to the manufacturer for quality control accountability.
3. Discarded, because it does not meet JCAHO policy regarding the packaging of commercially prepared items.
4. Sent to the hospital quality improvement committee for evaluation.

63. In a determination of the shelf life of a sterilized item, factors to be considered include the:
    1. Weight of the item, the size of the item, and the intended use of the item.
    2. Method of sterilization, the composition of the item, and the average length of time before item use.
    3. Dimensions of the item, the date on which the item was sterilized, and the method of sterilization.
    4. Packaging materials used, storage area conditions, and how many times the item is handled before use.

64. When positioning a patient on the transportation vehicle after carpal tunnel release under local anesthesia, the perioperative nurse ensures that the operative wrist is:
    1. Lowered to allow increased blood flow to the site and decrease potential for infection.
    2. Elevated to increase venous return and decrease swelling.
    3. Placed across the chest so that the hand can be easily observed during transfer.
    4. Held level to minimize circulatory compromise.

65. Avoiding or minimizing cardiovascular and respiratory compromise is a goal for a patient undergoing local anesthesia. Intraoperative evaluation can best be accomplished by:
    1. Monitoring the local anesthetic given, electrocardiography, pulse oximetry, and recording the patient's vital signs every 15 minutes.
    2. Checking the patient's chart for allergies, ensuring availability of oxygen in the OR, pulse oximetry, and obtaining an accurate blood-loss estimate.
    3. Calculating the total anesthetic dose, monitoring the physiological and psychosocial status, and ensuring that emergency equipment is available.
    4. Reviewing the patient's history, assessing breath sounds, and noting the time when local anesthesia is administered.

66. When formulating the nursing care plan, the perioperative nurse should be aware that the plan of care should:
    1. Reflect current nursing practice.
    2. Be left open to allow for each nurse to individualize patient care.
    3. Indicate how the action is adapted to a specific patient.
    4. Have a specific goal outlined for each physician order.

67. A patient undergoing a breast biopsy under local anesthesia of 1% lidocaine with epinephrine develops nausea, palpitations, and tachycardia. These signs are most likely a symptom of:
    1. Apprehension due to the possibility of an unfavorable diagnosis.
    2. Lack of adequate emotional support by the nurse.
    3. Hypersensitivity or toxicity.
    4. The cardiotonic effect of epinephrine.

68. A quality improvement program should be:
    1. Determined by a consensus of staff.
    2. Uniform for all clinical areas.
    3. A reflection of ideal nursing practice.
    4. Based on established standards.

69. Which of the following situations best illustrates the implementation phase of the nursing process?
    1. Documenting nursing care activities to promote continuity of care.
    2. Providing a mechanism for peer review in the OR.
    3. Checking records to determine the surgeon's preference for suture material.
    4. Reviewing the results of preoperative laboratory work.

70. A patient who is scheduled for a radical nephrectomy is 62 inches (157 cm) tall and weighs 180 lb (81.6 kg). For this patient, which one of the following is the most critical intraoperative nursing diagnosis?
    1. The patient is free from signs and symptoms of electrical injury.
    2. The patient is free from signs and symptoms of radiation injury.
    3. The patient is free of signs and symptoms of injury related to positioning.
    4. The patient is free of signs and symptoms of infection.

71. While observing surgery, a medical student who is wearing unsterile surgical attire accidentally brushes against the first assistant's sleeve. In this situation, the perioperative nurse's immediate action should be to:
    1. Tell the first assistant to stop operating and to change their sterile gown.
    2. Call attention to the break in aseptic technique and obtain a sterile sleeve for the first assistant.
    3. Tell the medical student to be more careful and to put on a sterile gown.
    4. Reprimand the medical student for carelessness and for inattention to the sterile field.

72. To evaluate kidney function after a blood transfusion reaction, the most appropriate intraoperative nursing action is to:
    1. Monitor the patient's cardiopulmonary response.
    2. Increase IV fluids to increase urine output.
    3. Save all transfusion bags and send these to the PACU with the patient.
    4. Send a urine sample to the laboratory for urinalysis.

73. Which of the following factors must be considered when applying and inflating a pneumatic tourniquet?
    1. Length of surgery, type of procedure, estimated blood loss, and presence of reflexes.
    2. Patient's age, physical status, and vascular supply to the extremity.
    3. Length of surgery, patient's age, cardiac output, and degree of muscular development in the legs.
    4. Size of extremity, presence of reflexes, cardiac output, and length of surgery.

74. When the phacoemulsification process is used to extract a cataract, the:
    1. Posterior lens of the eye is removed.
    2. Anterior lens of the eye is left in place.
    3. Entire lens of the eye is removed.
    4. Posterior lens of the eye is left in place.

75. The primary purpose of applying intermittent pressure to the eye following retrobulbar block injection is to:
    1. Decrease intraocular pressure.
    2. To aid in diffusion of the anesthetic agent.
    3. Prevent a reaction to the anesthetic agent.
    4. Decrease facial edema.

76. The planning phase of the nursing process is characterized by activities such as:
    1. Putting identified interventions into practice.
    2. Using new data to reassess nursing actions and patient goals.
    3. Reviewing the patient record for data collection and data analysis.
    4. Establishing goals, priorities, and evaluation criteria.

77. A 74-year-old patient is scheduled for an exploratory laparotomy. The nursing diagnosis, "The patient is at or returning to normothermia at the conclusion of the immediate portoperative period," is made. In developing a perioperative care plan for this patient, which one of the following should the perioperative nurse include?
    1. Provide the anesthesia provider with a blood/fluid warmer.
    2. Increase the operating room's ambient temperature to 80° F-85° F.
    3. Provide the surgeon with extra drape sheets for thermal insulation.
    4. Place antiembolism stockings on the patient's legs to improve circulation.

78. When instructing in the technique of instilling eyedrops, a perioperative nurse should tell the patient to:
    1. Look downward, then pull gently outward on the lower lid to form a receptacle for the medication.
    2. Recline, hyperextend the head, and open the eye very wide.
    3. Hyperextend the head and tilt the head to the side.
    4. Look upward, then pull gently outward on the lower lid to form a receptacle for the medication.

79. An effective operating room ventilation system should provide air exchanges at a minimum rate of:
    1. 8 per hour.
    2. 15 per hour.
    3. 20 per hour.
    4. 25 per hour.

80. When a carbon dioxide laser is to be used for a laser bronchoscopy, fire safety procedures begin with:
    1. Applying a damp head wrap to protect the patient.
    2. Placing wet drapes around the operative site.
    3. Draping the overhead suspension table with

damp drapes.
4. Shoulder draping to contain loose monitoring lines.

81. Due to cardiac irregularities during surgery, a patient is transferred postoperatively to the coronary care unit. In this situation, the primary responsibility of the perioperative nurse would be to:
   1. Call a member of the clergy to be with the patient's family.
   2. Make sure that the physician speaks to the patient's family.
   3. Wait until the prognosis is confirmed before speaking with the patient's family.
   4. Ensure that the patient's family is informed of the transfer.

82. A patient's nursing diagnosis is, "The patient is free from signs and symptoms of electrical injury." To evaluate the effect of the perioperative nurse's actions, documentation should include:
   1. The type of active electrode used, and the last check by biomedical personal.
   2. Assessing the patient's skin for signs of pallor.
   3. Patient's skin condition, ESU brand name, and placement of dispersive electrode.
   4. Assessing the patient skin for reaction from ESU and prep solution.

83. Use of metal knee crutch stirrups for lithotomy position has the potential for causing compromise to which nerve?
   1. Gluteal.
   2. Popliteal.
   3. Femoral.
   4. Peroneal.

84. While being transported to the PACU, a 19-year-old patient who received 10 mg of midazolam (Versed) during ambulatory rhinoplasty becomes cyanotic and unresponsive. The perioperative nurse suspects midazalom overdose and anticipates administration of:
   1. Atropine to increase the heart rate.
   2. Oxygen at 4 L/min via nasal cannula until voluntary respiration returns.
   3. Naloxone (Narcan) to reverse the effects of midazolam.
   4. Assisted ventilation until voluntary respiration returns.

85. According to AORN recommended practices, the perioperative nurse's care of patients receiving local anesthesia should include:
   1. Documenting all aspects of the surgical procedure being performed.
   2. Monitoring the patient's physiological and psychosocial status throughout the procedure.
   3. Talking to the patient and reassuring them throughout the entire the procedure.
   4. Maintaining the room temperature at 68° F to ensure a comfortable environment.

86. To effectively provide continuity of care postoperatively, an appropriate perioperative nursing action is to:
   1. Communicate any special patient needs to the PACU prior to the start of the procedure.
   2. Assign an orderly to transfer the patient to the PACU along with the patient's chart.
   3. Inform the charge nurse of special needs and ask that they communicate to the PACU.
   4. Complete all documentation of the OR record and send to PACU with the patient.

87. A perioperative nurse who is a member of the OR product evaluation committee is evaluating surgical masks, which also will be used by three other departments. Criteria used for the selection process includes all except:
   1. Cost.
   2. Efficiency.
   3. Color.
   4. Quality.

88. A young male trauma patient is admitted to the emergency department with no identification. The patient dies soon after arrival without ever regaining conscious. This patient does not meet the criteria for organ donation, because:
   1. The exact age of the patient is unknown.
   2. A history cannot be obtained.
   3. A valid donor card has not been found.
   4. No one may give consent for an unknown.

89. Managing the patient's anxiety by providing time and an opportunity for talking about fears and feelings is an example of:
   1. Assessment.
   2. Planning.
   3. Implementation.
   4. Evaluation.

90. Before the surgical procedure begins, a perforation is noticed in the scrub nurse's glove. The scrub nurse decides to change the glove using the closed-glove technique. A correct statement regarding the closed-glove technique is that this:

1. Should be used only when the gown and glove are first donned.
2. Is preferred over the open-glove method for subsequent gloving.
3. Can be used at any time during the surgical procedure.
4. Should be used by each surgical team member.

91. The surgeon performing a left carpal tunnel release under local anesthesia administers 5 cc of 1% lidocaine via infiltration into the incision site. In addition to route, dosage, and time of administration, accurate documentation would include which additional information about the local agent?
    1. Lot number.
    2. Potential side effects.
    3. Expiration date.
    4. Adverse effects.

92. When preparing for the possibility of malignant hyperthermia, which of the following approaches would be most effective to ensure that perioperative nursing staff are able to take appropriate actions?
    1. Delegate all responsibility for the recognition and treatment of malignant hyperthermia in the OR setting to the anesthesia personnel present.
    2. Require that selected perioperative staff members read professional journal articles related to malignant hyperthermia, and present a brief unit in-service review on the topic.
    3. Prepare malignant hyperthermia protocol for the OR that outlines perioperative nurse preparations, and review this protocol periodically with the OR staff.
    4. Require that all perioperative nurses attend an emergency in-service review pertaining to the risks of general anesthesia and malignant hyperthermia.

93. A perioperative nurse who is circulating on a routine exploratory laparotomy notices a blood-soaked laparotomy sponge on the floor. In response to this finding, the nurse should:
    1. Cover the sponge with an impervious towel and pick it up at the end of the case.
    2. Pick up the sponge with an impervious towel and spray the immediate area with a disinfectant.
    3. Cover the sponge with a towel, spray the towel with a disinfectant, and pick it up once the case has been completed.
    4. Pick up the sponge with gloved hands and clean the area using a facility-approved agent.

94. When the CO_2 laser is used, measures for patient safety should include:
    1. Covering the patient's eyes with a method approved by the laser safety officer.
    2. Using alcohol as an antiseptic prep solution.
    3. Removing all smoke evacuators from the room.
    4. Using bright, reflective instruments of the surgeons choice on the procedure.

95. According to AORN recommended practices, OR attire worn by the OR team should be changed:
    1. At the conclusion of each case.
    2. When it is visibly soiled or wet.
    3. Upon leaving the OR for lunch.
    4. At the conclusion of a contaminated case.

96. A program for monitoring exposure to ethylene oxide (EO) include all except:
    1. Compliance with OSHA regulations.
    2. Documentation of EO environmental monitoring.
    3. Adhering to JCAHO standards.
    4. Providing current information to each worker.

97. For employees exposed to ethylene oxide, the maximum permissible exposure in an 8-hour period is:
    1. 0.5 parts per million.
    2. 3 parts per million.
    3. 5 parts per million.
    4. 8 parts per million.

98. After the OR has been set up for a surgical procedure and the patient has arrived in the holding area, the surgery is delayed 2 hours. In accordance with AORN recommended practices, the perioperative nurse should:
    1. Close the OR door and tape it shut until the patient is brought in.
    2. Continuously monitor the sterile area for possible contamination.
    3. Refer to the established policy of the JCAHO.
    4. Cover the sterile supplies, using good aseptic technique.

99. Which of the following best describes patient positioning for a thoracotomy?
    1. Prone with arms extended over head.
    2. Supine with arms extended at 90 degrees.
    3. Jackknife and in reverse Trendelenburg.
    4. On unaffected side with a pillow between the knees.

100. During the preoperative assessment, a patient reports an allergy to shellfish and to IVP contrast media. Based on this information, the perioperative nurse should recognize the need to prep with:
    1. A antiseptic agent.
    2. A mild detergent.
    3. The surgeon's preference.
    4. A povidone/iodine solution.

101. In the evaluation of reusable gowns and drapes, primary consideration is given to:
    1. Availability in a variety of sizes.
    2. Patching ability.
    3. Barriers to microorganisms.
    4. Preshrinking of the fabric.

102. The perioperative nurse prepares to use a tourniquet and notices that the cuff is soiled. In response to this observation, the most appropriate action would be to:
    1. Put the soiled cuff back and use another.
    2. Wear gloves when applying the cuff.
    3. Wrap the arm with extra padding.
    4. Clean the cuff with a disinfectant.

103. For a total joint replacement, the surgeon ordered a Brand X implant, which arrives sterile and ready to use. During the procedure, the surgeon decides to use Brand Y because it will provide a better fit for the patient. The Brand Y implant is available but is not sterile. According to the AORN recommended practices, the nurse should:
    1. Sterilize the Brand Y implant, using an EO sterilization cycle and be completely aerated.
    2. Insist that the surgeon use the prepackaged Brand X implant which is already sterile.
    3. Flash the Brand Y implant with a biological indicator and wait for the results before using.
    4. Offer the surgeon other sterilized joint replacement implant choices.

104. A patient who has just been transferred to the OR bed for a cesarean section should be positioned supine with:
    1. Padding under the left hip.
    2. The head elevated.
    3. The legs elevated.
    4. Padding under the right hip.

105. For a patient who will be undergoing a cone biopsy of the cervix, sufficient padding is placed between the lateral aspects of the knee and the stirrup bars to:
    1. Prevent injury to the ankles and feet.
    2. Prevent injury to the lateral popliteal nerves.
    3. Protect the patient from possible hip dislocation.
    4. Protect from pressure and contact with metal surface.

106. In the instruction of an 8-year-old child, reasonable grasp of the information can often be ensured by the use of:
    1. No instruction is needed.
    2. Audio/visual aids.
    3. Group lectures.
    4. Reading material.

107. During a total hip arthroplasty, patient identification is crucial prior to dispensing which of the following?
    1. Bone homograft.
    2. Antibiotics.
    3. Total hip prosthesis.
    4. Autologous blood transfusion.

108. Intraoperatively, the surgeon requests that cultures be taken and sent to microbiology for analysis. Which of the following statements correctly applies to this situation?
    1. The culture tube and swabs were opened at the beginning of the case.
    2. The circulating nurse swabs the area where cultures are being taken using aseptic technique.
    3. The scrub nurse hands the culture tube to the circulating nurse in a sterile towel from the field.
    4. The culture tube is cleaned with a germicide and placed in an impervious container.

109. A laparotomy sponge had been retained in a patient and is discovered 6 months after surgery. All sponge, instrument, and needle counts had been recorded as correct. As employees of the hospital, the scrub nurse and the circulating nurse were held to be liable under the:
    1. Respondant superior doctrine.

2. Captain of the Ship.
3. Independent contractor principle.
4. Borrowed servant rule.

110. Information on the intraoperative nursing record should include patient's skin condition, positioning devices and supports, site of the dispersive electrode, use of lasers, and any:
    1. Records of flash sterilization performed during the procedure.
    2. Reason for delay of starting the surgery.
    3. Significant or unusual occurrences.
    4. Incident reports filed regarding the procedure.

111. The scrub nurse's gloves become contaminated intraoperatively. To reglove without involving another team member, the most appropriate method would be to:
    1. Use the open-glove technique.
    2. Remove gown and gloves, then regown and reglove.
    3. Place another pair of gloves over the contaminated gloves.
    4. Use the closed-glove technique.

112. After a procedure, donor bone not used will be saved for possible use at a later time. Of the following, which is the most important documentation to be placed on the donor bone container(s) by the perioperative nurse?
    1. Bone identification number, expiration date, and procurement center.
    2. Expiration date, perioperative nurse's name, and name of donor.
    3. Procurement center, date of procurement, and type of bone.
    4. Name of donor, type of bone saved, and date.

113. Mr. K is scheduled for a right inguinal hernia repair under general anesthesia. Mr. K is 39 years old, weighs 180 pounds, and is in good health. Immediately after induction, the anesthetist notes that Mr. K develops tachycardia, skin mottling, elevated body temperatuare, and muscle rigidity. Malignant hyperthermia is suspected. The perioperative nurses' first response would be to:
    1. Communicate with the patient's family, giving a brief explanation of what is suspected and tell them that the surgeon will be out to talk with them.
    2. Communicate with the head nurse to relay information on the situation and the condition of the patient.
    3. Obtain the malignant hyperthermia cart and cooling equipment.
    4. Notify the laboratory that a blood gas will be sent.

114. According to AORN recommended practices, which of the following considerations is most important regarding the safe use of an x-ray intraoperatively?
    1. Leaded shields should be in place to protect the patient.
    2. Leaded shields absorb the total amount of ionizing rays.
    3. Direct x-ray produces scatter more radiation than fluoroscopy does.
    4. Scattered radiation is decreased during oblique angle x-rays.

115. During transfer from the operating room (OR) suite to the postanesthesia care unit (PACU), the patient position of choice would be based on which of the following factors?
    1. Established hospital protocol.
    2. Maintainance of respiration/circulation.
    3. Distance from OR suite to PACU.
    4. Physician's preference.

116. A perioperative nurse is assigned to monitor a patient receiving moderate sedation/analgesia. At a minimum the RN should be competent in:
    1. Pharmacology.
    2. Starting an IV.
    3. Basic life support.
    4. Age-appropriate needs.

117. With regard to human immunodeficiency virus (HIV) testing associated with harvesting of bone for banking, a living donor must understand that:
    1. This test will be required 6 months prior to the bone harvesting procedure.
    2. A test will be done after donation and the tissue quarantined for at least 180 days.
    3. This test is not necessary because bone does not transmit HIV.
    4. This test will be administered only if the donor is considered a high-risk donor.

118. Postoperative instructions for a laser tonsillectomy patient should include which of the following?
    1. Increase diet from liquids, to soft, to normal the following day.
    2. Resume normal activity after 1 to 2 days.
    3. Avoid citrus fruits and dairy products.
    4. Reduce oral fluid intake.

119. A solution of 2% glutaraldehyde is categorized as which of the following types of disinfectant?
    1. High-level.
    2. Critical-level.
    3. Low-level.
    4. Intermediate-level.

120. The perioperative nurse converses periodically with the patient during a procedure being performed under moderate sedation/analgesia to verify level of consciousness. This practice represents which phase of the nursing process?
    1. Assessment.
    2. Planning.
    3. Implementation.
    4. Evaluation.

121. In order to reduce bacterial growth and suppress static electricity within the OR, the ideal humidity range should be:
    1. 20%-30%.
    2. 30%-40%.
    3. 40%-50%.
    4. 50%-60%.

122. "The omission to do something which a reasonable person, guided by those ordinary considerations which ordinarily regulate human affairs, would do, or the doing of something which a reasonable and prudent person would not do" is the legal definition of:
    1. Liability.
    2. Negligence.
    3. Malpractice.
    4. Imprudence.

123. Authoritative statements that describe the responsibilities for which nursing practitioners are accountable are called:
    1. Policies.
    2. Protocols.
    3. Guidelines.
    4. Standards.

124. In evaluating a product for possible purchase, which of the following is the most important?
    1. Safety of product.
    2. Cost of product.
    3. Need for product.
    4. User preference.

125. In using cricoid pressure during the induction of anesthesia, it is most important to:
    1. Document anoxic episodes.
    2. Inform the anesthesiologist of any difficulty.
    3. Maintain pressure until intubation is completed.
    4. Observe for the presence of gag reflexes.

126. During intraoperative monitoring of a healthy 36-year-old patient undergoing a breast biopsy under local anesthesia receiving moderate sedation/analgesia, the perioperative nurse should prepare to document:
    1. Oxygen saturation, temperature, and pulse.
    2. Blood pressure, and heart rate, and oxygen saturation.
    3. Temperature, pulse rate, and respirations.
    4. Electrocardiogram, blood pressure, and temperature.

127. Before transporting a trauma patient from the operating room to the intensive care unit, the perioperative nurse should have available:
    1. Oxygen equipment, an electrocardiogram monitor, and an arterial line.
    2. A Swan\Ganz catheter tray, a respirator, and an autotransfusion collection device.
    3. An intracranial pressure monitor, a patient-controlled analgesia pump, and a blood warmer.
    4. A tracheostomy tray, a peritoneal lavage set, and a sequential compression device.

128. Following an appendectomy, a blistered area is noted on the left thigh of the patient. In addition to documenting the finding, the perioperative nurse should:
    1. Check the hypothermia unit for any signs of malfunction.
    2. Apply a thin coating of antibiotic ointment to the affected area.
    3. Check the preoperative assessment for documentation of any allergies.
    4. Remove the ESU from service and save the active and dispersive electrode devices.

129. Four laparoscopic tubal ligations have been scheduled for the same day. One of the four available laparoscopes is contaminated during the preparation for the second tubal ligation. The laparoscopes will not withstand steam sterilization. In this situation, what would be the most appropriate course of action?
    1. Fill out an incident report noting deviation of standard of care, and soak the contaminated laparoscope in a high-level disinfectant for 20 minutes prior to use on the fourth patient.

2. Inform the surgeon, fill out an incident report noting deviation of standard of care, high-level disinfect the scope and/or try and borrow a sterile scope from another facility.
3. Inform the fourth patient that her tubal ligation cannot be done due to the lack of sterile equipment.
4. Sterilize the contaminated laparoscope using ethylene oxide, omit the aeration cycle, and rinse with sterile water.

130. After a patient has been repositioned, the surgeon repeatedly requests that the electrosurgical unit power be increased. The circulating nurse should:
   1. Inspect the dispersive electrode for full surface contact with the patient.
   2. Advance the setting and document on the OR record.
   3. Remove the ESU and send it to biomedical engineering.
   4. Offer a new active electrode handpiece and connect it to the same unit.

131. The x-ray technologist transports the C-arm from the storage room outside the operating room, into the operating room for a scheduled procedure. The circulating nurse should stop the technologist at the operating room entrance to:
   1. Inspect the machine for soilage, recognizing that disinfecting and damp dusting were done prior to storage.
   2. Advise the technologist to damp dust the machine using a facility-approved agent before entering the room.
   3. Inspect the machine for soilage and drape with a sterile C-arm drape before entry.
   4. Advise the technologist to damp dust the machine using a disinfectant after entering the room.

132. A patient undergoing abdominal hysterectomy has a hemoglobin value of 10g/dl and a hematocrit of 30%. Intraoperatively, the perioperative nurse notices 600 cc of bloody fluid in the suction canister. In this situation, the nurse would do all of the following except:
   1. Alert the surgeon and anesthesia care provider to the 600 cc of bloody fluid in the suction canister.
   2. Ask the scrub nurse how much irrigation has been used and subtract this amount from the 600 cc to estimate the partial blood loss.
   3. Weigh the soiled sponges to calulate the blood loss from the sponges.
   4. Obtain the crash cart, hang the blood expanders, and prepare paperwork for blood typing and cross-match.

133. Studies have shown the simplest and least irritating method of hair removal is accomplished by:
   1. Depilatories.
   2. Clippers.
   3. Razor.
   4. Waxing.

134. The correct protocol for assisted-gowning and gloving is:
   1. Using aseptic technique, open the sterile gown and gloves on a separate surface.
   2. Open the sterile gown and gloves on the back table, and have the incoming team member gown and glove themselves.
   3. Open the gown and gloves on the back table, and permit the scrub nurse to gown and glove the incoming team member.
   4. Ask the circulating nurse to first gown and glove and then assist the incoming team member.

135. A nursing care plan for geriatric patients undergoing surgical intervention may be:
   1. The patient is free from signs and symptoms of postoperative falls.
   2. The patient is at risk for decreased ability to hear verbal instructions.
   3. The patient is at risk for emotional and psychological stress.
   4. The patient is free from signs and symptoms of infection.

136. For sterilization of implantable medical devices the AORN recommended practices recommend:
   1. Sterilize then quarantine the implantable device and await the outcome of biological monitoring.
   2. Releasing the implant before the results of the biological monitoring device is known, then report the results to the surgeon as soon as the results are available.
   3. Flash sterilizing the implantable device for 10 minutes in a steam sterilizer with a biological monitoring device and use immediately.
   4. Flash sterilizing the implant for 3 minutes with a biological monitoring device and use immediately.

137. For personnel who will handle the transfer of the patient to the operating room bed, the perioperative

nurse should dispense protective gloves because:
1. The patient may not have been tested for human immunodeficiency virus (HIV).
2. The patient should be protected from cross-contamination.
3. Gloves are worn to reduce contamination of the hands of health care workers.
4. Gloves are considered personal protective equipment (PPE) and should be worn.

138. Which of the following events is the best indicator that the patient is ready to be moved to the postanesthesia care unit (PACU)?
   1. The surgeon indicates that the patient is ready.
   2. The nursing documentation is completed.
   3. The anesthesia care provider indicates that the patient is ready.
   4. The surgery is completed and the dressing is in place.

139. Before the surgical procedure begins, a sterile basin is opened and water is poured for the purpose of cleaning the powder from gloves. After everyone's gloves have been rinsed, the scrub nurse should:
   1. Retain the basin of water for possible glove-rinsing during the procedure.
   2. Place soiled instruments in the basin.
   3. Add antibiotic and additional water to the basin to use as a wound irrigation.
   4. Ask that the basin be removed from the sterile field.

140. A surgical mask should cover both mouth and nose, and it should be:
   1. Allowed to hang around the neck between procedures.
   2. Tied snugly with strings crossed.
   3. Changed after 2 hours of use.
   4. Removed and discarded after use handling only the ties.

141. During a total hip replacement, the perioperative nurse is exposed to bone cement (methyl methacrylate). The nurse should be concerned that exposure may cause:
   1. A chemical reaction with the sterile gloves.
   2. Irritation of the respiratory tract and eyes.
   3. A break in OR policies and procedures.
   4. Contamination of the sterile set-up.

142. Flexible endoscopes should be cleaned immediately after use according to manufacturers' written instructions that include:
   1. Flushing the internal channels with water and/or an enzymatic detergent.
   2. Soaking in an intermediate level disinfectant for 20 minutes before handling.
   3. Placed in an ultrasonic cleaner to assist in removing debris from crevices.
   4. Spraying with an enzymatic solution and transported to the decontamination area.

143. During an operative procedure, the gloves worn by the scrub nurse working within the sterile field become contaminated. In removing these gloves, the circulating nurse avoids pulling the cuff of the gown over the nurse's hand, because the:
   1. The stockinette cuff of the gown is considered unsterile.
   2. The sleeve of the gown may become contaminated in the process.
   3. Stockinette cuff can become contaminated during removal of the glove.
   4. The circulating nurse can contaminate their hands with the soiled glove.

144. After a patient has been positioned in the lateral position, the intraoperative nursing documentation should include identification of:
   1. Personnel who assisted with positioning.
   2. Potential skin and/or nerve problems.
   3. Patient positioning devices and supports.
   4. Nerves, muscles, or blood vessels injured during the procedure.

145. Correct placement of the patients arms when in the supine position include all of the following except:
   1. On arm boards, less than a 90-degree angle, with elbow padding applied.
   2. Secured to the OR bed with soft non-occlusive wrist restraints and elbow padding applied.
   3. At the patient's sides with palms supinated and tucked and the draw sheet over the arm.
   4. At the patient's sides with palms neutral against the body and fingers straight.

146. Documentation for a patient undergoing vaginal hysterectomy would identify the wound as:
   1. Contaminated.
   2. Dirty.
   3. Clean.
   4. Clean contaminated.

147. Which of the following perioperative nursing interventions is most effective for reducing the

possibility of contamination of the sterile field?
1. Consider the back of a wrap-around gown sterile.
2. Reposition the drapes if the patient is repositioned.
3. Place sterile drapes on patient, furniture, and equipment.
4. Use the double-glove method for all surgical procedures.

148. Halfway through a bilateral lower-extremity debridement and skin graft on a patient with third-degree burns, the surgeon requests that the drapes be repositioned farther apart to achieve better surgical access. According to AORN recommended practices, the scrub nurse's most appropriate action is to:
1. Move the drapes to best accommodate the surgeon's access to the surgical site.
2. Notify the surgeon that once the drapes are placed they should not be moved.
3. Request a laparotomy drape to re-drape the entire sterile field.
4. Use sterile towels to cover the edges of the original drapes.

149. A patient having a lymph node biopsy has tested seropositive for the HIV virus. On the record, the nurse would document:
1. HIV-positive.
2. AIDS patient.
3. Standard precautions noted for this patient.
4. Nothing specific to identify the patient's HIV status.

150. During an appendectomy, the scrub nurse assists the surgeon in collecting aerobic and anaerobic cultures of the peritoneal fluid. The perioperative nurse's first action after receiving the specimens from the scrub nurse should be to:
1. Don sterile gloves before handling the specimens.
2. Wipe the culture tubes with a chemical germicide.
3. Place the cultures a sterile container for transport.
4. Document pertinent information regarding the specimens.

151. The OR manager notices that the circulating nurse is wearing a turtleneck sweater under the regulation scrub attire, and directs the nurse to remove this turtleneck sweater. The manager makes this request because she realizes that:
1. The nurse had recently come from a room where the temperature was 18° C (65° F), and was still cold.
2. Clothing from home worn outside the surgical attire is prohibited unless approved by the infection control committee.
3. Clothing from home worn in the surgical suite must be completely contained or covered by the surgical scrub attire.
4. The nurse is wearing the turtleneck sweater in an effort to provide a comfortable environment.

152. Studies show that the lowest infection rates have been noted in surgical cases where patient body hair was:
1. Not removed.
2. Removed using a depilatory.
3. Cut with surgical clippers.
4. Shaved.

153. While setting up the sterile field before the patient entered the room, the scrub nurse notices a fly on the back table. The nurse would first destroy the fly and then:
1. Reglove and have the circulating nurse replace all opened sterile supplies on the back table.
2. Regown and reglove and proceed with setting up the back table.
3. Reglove and then cover the area of the sterile field on which the fly was observed.
4. Remove the entire back table setup and replace all opened sterile supplies.

154. When the scrub nurse working at the sterile field requests a mallet, the most appropriate way for the circulating nurse to transfer the instrument to the sterile field is to:
1. Place it in the middle of the back table.
2. Roll the mallet onto the mayo stand.
3. Drop the item into the basin of water.
4. Wait until the scrub nurse can take the item.

155. A large volume of surgical smoke could be generated by the electrosurgical unit during a reduction mammoplasty. To reduce the hazards associated with smoke plume the perioperative nurse could use all of the following except:
1. A smoke evacuation system.
2. Surgical filtration mask.
3. A respiratory evacuation system.
4. Wall suctions with in-line filters.

156. Which anesthetic agents are most likely to trigger a negative reaction in a patient with a family history of malignant hyperthermia undergoing a procedure using general anesthesia?
   1. An inhalational anesthtic and succinylcholine.
   2. Versed and Fentanyl.
   3. Diflorasone (Florone) and midazolam.
   4. Nitrous oxide and atropine.

157. What is the relationship between the weight of a bloody sponge and patient blood loss intraoperatively?
   1. 1 gm of weight equals 0.5 mL of blood loss.
   2. 1 gm of weight equals 1 mL of blood loss.
   3. 2 gm of weight equals 0.5 mL of blood loss.
   4. 2 gm of weight equals 1 mL of blood loss.

158. According to recent studies, the most important factor in preventing wound infection is:
   1. Surgical technique.
   2. Surgical hand scrubbing.
   3. Antibiotic prophylaxis.
   4. Surgical skin scrub.

159. The overall goal of asepsis in the surgical environment is:
   1. Minimize contamination of the surgical wound.
   2. Cleanliness and elimination of all infectious agents.
   3. Ensure no breaks in sterile technique.
   4. Guarantee pathogens do not harm the patient.

160. Which the following correctly describes personal protective equipment (PPE) by the Occupational Safety and Health Administration (OSHA) regulation established to prevent occupational exposure to bloodborne pathogens?
   1. Masks, gowns, eye protection, and fluid-proof shoe covers.
   2. Scrub attire, hats, sterile gloves, and face shields.
   3. Sterile gowns, gloves, head coverings, and lab coats.
   4. Disposable gowns, gloves, and head and foot coverings.

161. The most commonly accepted recommendations for flash sterilization parameters are established by which agency?
   1. Association for Practitioners in Infection Control (APIC).
   2. Joint Commission on Accreditation of Healthcare Organizations (JCAHO).
   3. National Institute for Occupational Safety and Health (NIOSH).
   4. Association for the Advancement of Medical Instrumentation (AAMI).

162. The perioperative nurse would notify the anesthesia provider if a patient's potassium level is 6.1 mEq/L on arrival in the holding area, because this finding places the patient at risk for:
   1. Increased cellular uptake.
   2. Renal failure.
   3. Gastrointestinal losses.
   4. Muscle cramps.

163. The appropriate sequence of steps for cleaning instruments in a washer/decontaminator may include:
   1. Washing, rinsing with distilled water, drying, sterilizing, and rinsing.
   2. Rinsing, enzaymatic soak, washing, hot water rinse, chemical germicide rinse, and drying.
   3. Sorting, rinsing, washing, ultrasonic cleaning, drying, and sterilizing.
   4. Sorting, washing, rinsing with tap water, drying, and processing.

164. Criteria for the care of surgical patients with a latex allergy may include all except:
   1. Latex allergy questionnaire.
   2. Latex-safe cart.
   3. Latex-safe policies and procedures.
   4. Latex free designated OR.

165. When choosing a pneumatic tourniquet cuff for a patient, the perioperative nurse selects a cuff:
   1. That is narrow to expose as much of the limb as possible.
   2. With adequate length to overlap at least 3 inches but not more than 6 inches.
   3. Based on the patient's age and blood pressure.
   4. By considering the average length of the planned surgical procedure.

166. When adding a basin to the sterile field, the perioperative nurse notes water droplets on the inside of the basin. The basin is considered:
   1. Unsterile without consideration of the wrap material.
   2. Sterile since the condensation occurred after sterilization.
   3. Unsterile unless wrapped in water-impermeable film.
   4. Sterile since the wrap material is absorbent and water-impermeable.

167. When a pneumatic tourniquet is used, documentation should include all of the following except:
   1. Cuff location, pressure, and identification number of specific tourniquet.
   2. Inflation and deflation times, and skin protection used under tourniquet.
   3. Size of cuff, identification number of tourniquet, and last maintenance check.
   4. Assessment of extremity and identification of person who applied the cuff.

168. During the fibroplastic phase of wound healing, there is evidence of:
   1. Exudate containing blood, lymph, and fibrin.
   2. Epithelial cells, collagen synthesis, and wound contraction.
   3. Scar tissue formed with new collagen produced.
   4. Separation of layers of the surgical wound.

169. To provide optimal care for a patient receiving intravenous conscious sedation, the perioperative nurse arranges for:
   1. Monitored anesthesia care to manage the patient
   2. A CRNA to manage the patient receiving conscious sedation.
   3. A second registered nurse to manage the patient receiving conscious sedation.
   4. The procedure to be carried out in the ambulatory surgery center.

170. When combined, the most effective antimicrobial surgical hand scrub agents include:
   1. Iodophors and triclosan.
   2. Alcohol and iodophors.
   3. Chlorhexidine gluconate and alcohol.
   4. Triclosan and chlorhexidine gluconate.

171. All processed sterile items for the OR come from the central service area. Frequently, items are needed immediately but the central service technician cannot seem to understand that these requests should take priority. Which of the following would be most beneficial in solving this problem?
   1. Request that the technician's shift be changed so that he/she will be working during the "slack" hours.
   2. Counsel the technician and tell him/her that disciplinary action may be taken.
   3. Have the technician spend some time in the operating room observing procedures.
   4. Request that the technician be assigned to a less critical area of central service.

172. You are on a committee responsible for the needle count policy in your operating room. Your primary rationale for implementing the count is:
   1. Patient and personnel safety.
   2. Inventory control.
   3. Effective cost analysis.
   4. Legal accountability.

173. Which one of the following is an incorrect practice when a patient is transported via a transportation vehicle?
   1. Attach tubes and drainage devices to maintain integrity and function.
   2. Push the transport vehicle with the patient feet first.
   3. Use the safety straps on the transportation vehicle.
   4. Place the intravenous containers at the head of the vehicle.

174. A patient is undergoing a choledochostomy to relieve obstruction. After all stones are removed, the common duct is thoroughly flushed with:
   1. A 10% glycerin solution.
   2. A 0.9% saline solution.
   3. An antibiotic solution.
   4. A lactated ringers solution.

175. Equipment and supplies necessary to carry out standard precautions should be available to operating room personnel to minimize the risk of exposure in which of the following situations?
   1. Patients that have a history of HIV.
   2. Cases in which patients have a history of hepatitis C.
   3. All cases and all patients regardless of their history.
   4. Cases in which patients have a history of pulmonary TB.

176. When opening sterile supplies to be dispensed to the sterile field, which of the following actions by a perioperative nurse would demonstrate proper aseptic technique?
   1. Flipping the contents of a sterile package onto the back table.
   2. Checking a dropped package for any signs of moisture before dispensing.
   3. Checking the sterile package for perforations and process indicators.
   4. Sliding a pair of sterile gloves out of the outer wrapper.

177. Before the start of the first case of the day, the perioperative nurse should first:
   1. Damp dust all horizontal surfaces in the OR.
   2. Ask housekeeping to terminally clean the OR.
   3. Visually inspect the OR for cleanliness and then open sterile supplies.
   4. Note that the OR was terminally cleaned the evening before.

178. Additional clamps are required during a surgical procedure. Before dispensing the clamps to the sterile field, the perioperative nurse should check the package integrity, the chemical process indicator, and the:
   1. Date of sterilization.
   2. Expiration date.
   3. Load control number.
   4. Rotation date.

179. Postoperative transfer of a patient with known blood-borne pathogens requires the implementation of:
   1. Reverse isolation.
   2. Standard precautions.
   3. Transmission based precautions.
   4. Universal precautions.

180. One method to prevent venous stasis intraoperatively is to:
   1. Use special pressure stockings.
   2. Pad pressure points.
   3. Apply a pulse oximeter.
   4. Use an arterial Doppler monitor.

181. An infection control practitioner is inspecting for breaks in the application of standard precautions. The most serious violation of standard precautions would be a:
   1. Nurse without a cover gown outside the OR.
   2. Scrub nurse without protective eyewear.
   3. Nurse starting an IV line without double-gloving.
   4. Scrub nurse placing needles in an impervious color-coded receptacle.

182. The radiation-attenuating gloves used in fluoroscopy procedures block radiation dosage by which percentage?
   1. 20%
   2. 30%
   3. 40%
   4. 50%

183. A patient is scheduled for debridement of an infected wound. An orthopedic case is scheduled to follow this case, but the orthopedic surgeon refuses to do that case following a known contaminated case. In this situation, the best response by the perioperative nurse would be to inform the orthopedic surgeon that:
   1. Use of a high-level germicide will kill all microorganisms, so that the OR where the infectious case was treated is now clean and ready to use.
   2. The orthopedic case can proceed without delay, because case cleanup is the same for all cases, with standard precautions being followed.
   3. The orthopedic case should not proceed in an OR where an infectious case has just been performed.
   4. Microorganisms move independently, so that airing time is required in the OR where the contaminated case was treated.

184. When surgery is completed, the anesthesia provider states that the patient must remain intubated while in the PACU. In arranging for the patient's care, the perioperative nurse:
   1. Alerts the PACU that the patient will arrive intubated and may need respiratory therapy.
   2. Alerts the radiology department that the patient will remain intubated in the PACU.
   3. Notifies the respiratory therapist concerning the time the patient should be extubated.
   4. Notifies the surgeon and the PACU to extubate the patient when appropriate.

185. During the skin preparation of a patient undergoing a colostomy revision, the perioperative nurse will prep in a:
   1. Circular motion, progressing from the center of the anticipated incision to the periphery, prepping the colostomy site last.
   2. Back-and-forth motion, progressing from the colostomy site out to the periphery.
   3. Circular motion, progressing from the colostomy site out to the periphery.
   4. Back-and-forth motion, progressing from the center of the anticipated incision to the periphery prepping the colostomy site last.

186. The most important reason that movement of personnel during invasive procedures should be kept to a minimum is to reduce:
   1. Noise level.
   2. Airborne contamination.

3. Contamination of sterile team members.
4. Interference with anesthesia provider.

187. A perioperative nurse observes the door from the OR to the corridor opening and closing several times during a procedure. This is a violation of the traffic pattern rationale concerned with which of the following?
    1. The air pressure within each OR should be greater than that within the semi-restricted area.
    2. The potential for airborne contamination is enhanced by increased movement.
    3. Sterility is maintained when air pressure is lower in the OR than in the semi-restricted area.
    4. Bacteria counts rise sharply as air travels through the OR.

188. The degree of contamination with microorganisms and organic debris is known as:
    1. Bioshielding.
    2. Bioresistance.
    3. Biostate.
    4. Bioburden.

189. Which of the following is the currently accepted definition of sterility?
    1. Absense of resident and transient microbes.
    2. The complete elimination of all bioburden, including vegetative spores.
    3. The complete elimination of all forms of microbial life.
    4. Absence of infectious organisms.

190. There are three types of regulated waste generated by health care facilities. They include all of the following except:
    1. Radioactive waste.
    2. Hazardous chemical waste.
    3. Potentially infective waste.
    4. Solid and liquid waste.

191. The most important consideration in the design of the hat or hood should be:
    1. The prevention of the transmission of microorganisms.
    2. The use of skullcaps to cover all of the hair and scalp.
    3. The dispersal of microbes is minimized.
    4. The ease of donning the head covering.

192. According to the AORN recommended practices, the accepted methods for scrubbed personnel to recap a needle are to use a:
    1. Two-handed technique or ask the surgeon to recap the needle.
    2. Two-handed technique or a mechanical device.
    3. One-handed technique or wear two pairs of gloves.
    4. One-handed technique or a mechanical device.

193. All of the following are desirable characteristics of an antimicrobial agent for surgical scrubbing except:
    1. Fast-acting.
    2. Broad-spectrum.
    3. Non-irritating.
    4. No residual effect.

194. An important consideration in the management of patient-contact materials for patients infected with methicillin-resistant *Staphylococcus aureus* (MRSA) is:
    1. Clean and disinfect all patient care equipment.
    2. Incinerating all patient-contaminated materials post procedure.
    3. Require OR personal involved with the patient to wear two pairs of gloves.
    4. Culture all OR personal to determine who is a carrier.

195. All of the following medications used in moderate sedation/analgesia are classified as opioids except:
    1. Meperidin.
    2. Naloxone.
    3. Fentanyl.
    4. Morphine sulfate.

196. Which of the following local anesthetics is an aminoester?
    1. Lidocaine (Xylocaine).
    2. Mepivacaine (Carbocaine).
    3. Bupivacaine (Marcaine).
    4. Tetracaine (Pontocaine).

197. One of the components of a program for environmental responsibility in the OR include:
    1. Reprocessing and reusing single-use items.
    2. Opening all supplies on the physician preference card.
    3. Use of a knee-operated faucet during the hand scrub.
    4. Sterilizing most equipment with ethylene oxide (EO).

198. Proper surgical attire for non-scrubbed personnel includes:
    1. Scrub pants and top laundered at home.
    2. Wearing a double surgical mask.
    3. Sterile single-use gloves.
    4. A long-sleeved jacket closed in front.

199. Contaminated sponges should be handled and disposed of according to guidelines established by:
    1. Joint Commission on Accreditation of Healthcare Organizations (JCAHO) and facility policies and procedures.
    2. JCAHO and Occupational Safety and Health Administration (OSHA).
    3. AORN recommended practices, OSHA, and facility policies and procedures.
    4. OSHA, JCAHO, and AORN recommended practices.

200. Instrument counts should be taken in all of the following situations except:
    1. Before all emergency procedures.
    2. Before the procedure to establish a baseline.
    3. Before wound closure begins.
    4. At the time of permanent relief.

APPENDIX II: ANSWER KEY TO PRACTICE QUESTIONS

QUESTION	ANSWER
1	2
2	1
3	3
4	2
5	2
6	3
7	2
8	2
9	1
10	1
11	2
12	2
13	1
14	1
15	2
16	4
17	3
18	4
19	3
20	3
21	3
22	4
23	4
24	3
25	2
26	4
27	1
28	3
29	1

QUESTION	ANSWER
30	1
31	2
32	3
33	4
34	1
35	3
36	3
37	4
38	4
39	4
40	4
41	3
42	2
43	4
44	1
45	1
46	2
47	1
48	2
49	3
50	4
51	2
52	4
53	1
54	2
55	3
56	4
57	4
58	2
59	4

QUESTION	ANSWER	QUESTION	ANSWER
60	3	100	1
61	4	101	3
62	1	102	4
63	4	103	3
64	2	104	4
65	3	105	4
66	1	106	2
67	3	107	3
68	4	108	4
69	1	109	1
70	3	110	3
71	2	111	1
72	4	112	1
73	2	113	3
74	3	114	1
75	2	115	2
76	1	116	3
77	1	117	2
78	4	118	3
79	2	119	1
80	2	120	3
81	4	121	4
82	3	122	3
83	4	123	4
84	3	124	1
85	2	125	3
86	4	126	2
87	3	127	1
88	2	128	4
89	2	129	2
90	1	130	1
91	4	131	2
92	3	132	4
93	4	133	2
94	1	134	3
95	2	135	4
96	3	136	1
97	1	137	3
98	1	138	3
99	4	139	4

QUESTION	ANSWER
140	4
141	2
142	1
143	1
144	3
145	3
146	4
147	3
148	2
149	4
150	2
151	3
152	1
153	4
154	4
155	3
156	1
157	2
158	1
159	2
160	1
161	4
162	2
163	2
164	4
165	2
166	1
167	3
168	2
169	3
170	3
171	3
172	4
173	4
174	2
175	3
176	4
177	1
178	1
179	2

QUESTION	ANSWER
180	1
181	2
182	4
183	2
184	1
185	1
186	2
187	1
188	4
189	3
190	4
191	3
192	4
193	4
194	1
195	2
196	4
197	3
198	4
199	3
200	1

APPENDIX III:

GLOSSARY OF TERMS

Accountable
The state of being answerable to self, patient, profession, and agency for nursing care given in the operating room.

Advance Directive
A patient's signed and witnessed directive regarding health care, life-sustaining, and end-of-life decisions.

Ambulatory Surgery
For purposes of this document, outpatient surgery, same-day surgery, day surgery, etc, are included in the term *ambulatory surgery*.

AORN, Association of periOperative Registered Nurses
AORN is the professional organization of perioperative registered nurses that supports registered nurses in achieving optimal outcomes for patients undergoing operative and other invasive procedures. (www.aorn.org)

AORN Standards, Recommended Practices, and Guidelines
As used in the Job Analysis, this term includes all sections of the *Standards, Recommended Practices, and Guidelines* published annually by AORN. The most current edition should be used at all times.

Assessment
Collecting data about a patient to determine the appropriate nursing diagnosis and expected outcomes. Includes patient's history and physical, vital signs, and all aspects of presenting condition. Assessment begins with data collection and ends with the formation of nursing diagnoses. Assessment is ongoing during the perioperative period (ie, includes preoperative, intraoperative, postoperative).

Association for the Advancement of Medical Instrumentation (AAMI)
An organization with the goal of increasing the understanding and beneficial use of medical instrumentation. AAMI is the primary source of consensus and timely information on medical instrumentation and technology and is the primary resource for the industry, the professions, and government for national and international standards. (www.aami.org)

Autonomy
In the context of health care, autonomy is the patient's self-determination or ability and power to make his or her own decisions regarding health care.

Centers for Disease Control and Prevention (CDC)
The federal government agency dedicated to monitoring disease and mortality and morbidity of patients in the United States. This agency sets guidelines on dealing with known or suspected diseases. The CDC serves as the national focus for developing and applying disease prevention and control, environmental health, and health promotion and education activities designed to improve the health of the people of the United States. (www.cdc.gov)

Certification
The documented validation of the professional achievement of identified standards of practice of an individual registered nurse providing patient care before, during, and after surgery.

Code of Ethics

Guidelines regarding professional behavior and ethical decision making developed by the American Nurses Association. AORN has developed "explications for perioperative nursing" for each statement in the ANA code.

Community Resources

Other agencies that the perioperative nurse may refer patients to for special needs (eg, American Cancer Society, American Heart Association, home health care agencies, social services, organ procurement agencies).

Competency

The knowledge, skills, and abilities necessary to fulfill assigned job functions.

Continuous Quality Assessment and Improvement

The continuous monitoring and evaluation of activities and services to improve the delivery of health care.

Continuum of Care

Care of patients undergoing operative or other invasive procedures is planned and implemented along a continuum—from the time the decision to undergo surgery is made, through the intraoperative period, and for an undetermined postoperative period until the patient's health status is improved or a specified health goal is reached.

Cultural Diversity

Perioperative nurses must be aware of the variety of backgrounds, beliefs, values, and ethnicity among patients. This diversity plays a major role in the communication efforts and actions of perioperative nurses. Every patient must be evaluated for individual cultural considerations in the perioperative setting.

Delegation

The transfer of responsibility for the performance of an activity from one individual to another while retaining accountability for the outcome.

Demonstration/Return Demonstration

The act of teaching that involves the visible, active demonstration of an activity, then involving the learner by having them demonstrate the identical activity back to the teacher.

Discharge Planning

The process of assessing the needs of patients for post-procedure care; developing a coordinated and multidisciplinary plan to provide the care required (including patient/family education, available services, and referral agencies and/or support groups); and evaluating the plan. The process begins before or on admission to the health care facility.

Documentation

The written record of nursing care including patient assessment, the actions taken as a result of that assessment, the plan of care developed and implemented, and the results of those actions. Documentation serves as the main, retrievable communication tool for the health care team.

Domain (related to certification)

A categorization of job responsibilities that includes the functions and tasks performed by perioperative nurses. Used for designing the certification examination.

Domain (related to the PNDS)

The four overall divisions of the conceptual framework of the *Perioperative Nursing Data Set.* All interventions and expected outcomes relate to one or more domain. The four domains are "Safety," "Physiologic Responses," "Behavioral Responses," and the "Health System."

Ergonomics

An applied science concerned with designing and arranging things (eg, furniture, equipment) so that people can use the items efficiently and safely.

Extraneous Objects

Considered to be all equipment and supplies in the operating room, other than the patient and the health care team members. Includes all devices used, attached to the patient, or available in the room.

Family

For purposes of this document, the terms *significant others* and *extended family* are included in the term *family*.

First Assistant (RN)

The RN first assistant (RNFA) at surgery collaborates with the surgeon and the health care team in performing a safe operation with optimal outcomes for the patient. The RNFA practices perioperative nursing and must have acquired the necessary knowledge, skills, and judgment specific to clinical practice. The RNFA practices in collaboration with and at the direction of the surgeon during the intraoperative phase of the perioperative experience. The RNFA does not concurrently function as a scrub nurse. (AORN's "Official Statement on RN First Assistants.")

Health Care Team
The providers of patient care services who are required to provide direct patient care to help the patient achieve a positive outcome. Support services include, but are not limited to, pharmacy, radiology, blood bank, housekeeping, etc.

Healthcare Insurance Portability and Accountability Act (HIPAA)
Legislation passed in 1996 that addresses various aspects of the use of patients' medical information, including confidentiality of patient information in the medical record, consent processes for access to patients' health information, and the right to sue the health plan provider.

Hyperthermia
See Malignant Hyperthermia

Hypothermia
A body temperature significantly below normal (ie, 98.6° F [37° C]). May be caused by the operating room environment (eg, room temperature, exposed skin) and can interfere with patient's maintenance of a normal physiological state.

Informed Consent
The patient's right to make his or her own informed decisions based on information regarding treatment options, including the benefits, expected outcomes, and risk and potential complications; right to refuse treatment; and decisions regarding participation in research studies.

Intervention (Nursing)
Action taken, based on patient assessment data, with the intention of achieving one or more expected patient outcome.

Intraoperative Phase
Begins when the patient is transferred to the operating room bed and ends when he/she is admitted to the postanesthesia care unit.

Jehovah's Witness
A religious order whose members do not believe in the value or accept the transfusion of blood or blood products.

Job Analysis
The CBPN Job Analysis describes the overall functions and responsibilities as well as the underlying knowledge and skills that are essential to ensure proficiency as a perioperative nurse.

Joint Commission on Accreditation of Healthcare Organizations (JCAHO)
The independent accrediting organization that designates acceptable patient care and evaluates health care facilities' abilities to adhere to specific guidelines (eg, documentation, processes, policies, procedures). (www.jcaho.org)

Knowledge
Defined as an organized body of information, usually of a factual or procedural nature, which, if applied, makes adequate performance of a job possible. Possession of knowledge does not ensure its proper application.

Malignant Hyperthermia
The rapid onset of extremely high fever with muscle rigidity, precipitated by exogenous agents in genetically susceptible people. Some anesthesia medications may induce this condition.

Minimally Invasive Surgery
Surgery not requiring traditional incisions (ie, performed through ports through which instrumentation are introduced).

Nonmaleficence
In the context of health care, acting in the best interest of the patient for the benefit of the patient.

North American Nursing Diagnosis Association (NANDA)
The group that has developed a list of 155 accepted nursing diagnoses to ensure that documentation in all areas of nursing use consistent, comparable terminology. (www.nanda.org)
Also see Perioperative Nursing Data Set.

Nursing Diagnosis
A statement derived from the nursing assessment data that provides the framework for nursing interventions that enable the patient to attain specific

desired outcomes. It is structured using standardized nursing nomenclature. *Also see NANDA and Perioperative Nursing Data Set.*

Nursing Process
The critical thinking a nurse uses to assess the health status of patients, identify problems, develop and implement plans of care, and evaluate the patients' responses to that care.

Occupational Safety and Health Administration (OSHA)
The federal government agency (a division of the US Department of Labor) that sets standards for and investigates the proper physical condition of working environments. OSHA's mission is to ensure safe and healthful workplaces in the United States. (www.osha.gov)

Outcome Criteria
Statements developed to identify the tasks or conditions to be implemented that will assist the patient in achieving the desired outcomes. Outcome criteria indicate an expected, measurable change in the patient's health status.

Patients' Rights
Every patient has the right to seek and receive health care regardless of his/her race, religion, or culture and with respect for the individual's self-image, privacy, and other such considerations, in accordance with the Patients' Bill of Rights.

***Perioperative Nursing Data Set* (PNDS)**
The structured and standardized vocabulary of perioperative nursing care, including perioperative nursing diagnoses, interventions, and outcome statements. This vocabulary, developed by AORN, has been recognized by the American Nurses Association as useful in clinical practice.

Perioperative Period
Time commencing with the decision for surgical intervention and ending with a follow-up home/clinic evaluation. This period includes the preoperative, intraoperative, and postoperative phases.

Plan of Care (or Care Plan)
A result of a systematic process of identifying expected patient outcomes and determining how to achieve them. It includes the list of interventions necessary to reach the expected outcome. The plan of care directs all nursing care activities related to each patient.

Postoperative Phase
Begins with admission to the postanesthesia care area and ends with the resolution of surgical sequelae.

Preoperative Phase
Begins when the decision for surgical intervention is made and ends with the transfer of the patient to the operating room bed.

Professional Achievement
The attainment of a measurable level of performance. In the context of CNOR certification, the level is set on a continuum between competency and excellence in perioperative nursing. Professional achievement affirms that the perioperative nurse demonstrates consistent application of the nursing process and the identified specialty standards of practice.

Regulatory and Voluntary Guidelines and Standards
CDC, JCAHO, HHS, and OSHA regulations and standards and federal, state, and local laws/regulations that govern practice.

Reportable Event
An event designated as serious enough (ie, causing actual or potential harm to a patient) that it is required to be reported to the US Food and Drug Administration.

Safe Environment
The setting in which the physical and psychological aspects of the environment are controlled for the purpose of presenting the least possible hazard to the patient, staff members, and community.

Significant Other
See Family

Skill
Defined as the proficient manual, verbal, or mental manipulation of data, people, or things. Skill embodies observable, quantifiable, and measurable performance parameters.

Standard Precautions
As used in the Job Analysis, this term refers to the standard and transmission-based precautions policies and procedures as developed by the CDC and OSHA.

Supervision
The active process of directing, guiding, and influencing the outcome of an individual's performance of an activity.

Support Services
Pharmacy, radiology, blood bank, laboratories, environmental services (ie, housekeeping), biomedical engineering, etc.

Surgical Intervention
The patient's experiences during the preoperative, intraoperative, and postoperative phases including the technical aspects and anatomical approach.

Surgical Procedure
The technical aspects and anatomical approach used during surgical intervention.

Teaching/Learning Theories and Techniques
Those aids and methods that facilitate learning (eg, audiovisual tools, return demonstration, adult learning principles).

Transfer
Moving a patient from one place to another (eg, to or from a bed or stretcher, the stretcher to OR bed.).

Transport
Moving a patient via a device (wheelchair, stretcher, wagon).

Unlicensed Assistive Personnel
Individuals who are trained to function in an assistive role to the registered nurse in providing patient care activities as delegated by, and under the supervision of, the registered nurse.

INDEX